Edition

3

Laboratory Manual for

Clinical Kinesiology and Anatomy

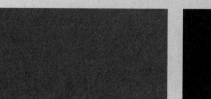

Edition 3

Laboratory Manual for

Clinical Kinesiology and Anatomy

Lynn S. Lippert, PT, MS

Program Director, Retired
Mt. Hood Community College
Gresham, Oregon

Mary Alice Duesterhaus Minor, PT, MS

Clinical Assistant Professor
Clarkson University
Potsdam, New York

F.A. Davis Company • Philadelphia

F. A. Davis Company
1915 Arch Street
Philadelphia, PA 19103
www.fadavis.com

Printed in the United States of America

Last digit indicates print number: 10 9 8 7 6 5 4 3 2 1

Acquisitions Editor: Melissa A. Duffield
Manager of Content Development: George W. Lang
Developmental Editor: Karen E. Williams
Art and Design Manager: Carolyn O'Brien

As new scientific information becomes available through basic and clinical research, recommended treatments and drug therapies undergo changes. The author(s) and publisher have done everything possible to make this book accurate, up to date, and in accord with accepted standards at the time of publication. The author(s), editors, and publisher are not responsible for errors or omissions or for consequences from application of the book, and make no warranty, expressed or implied, in regard to the contents of the book. Any practice described in this book should be applied by the reader in accordance with professional standards of care used in regard to the unique circumstances that may apply in each situation. The reader is advised always to check product information (package inserts) for changes and new information regarding dose and contraindications before administering any drug. Caution is especially urged when using new or infrequently ordered drugs.

To students who desire to understand so as to help others.

MADM

■ ■ ■ Preface to Third Edition

The major change to this third edition of *Laboratory Manual for Clinical Kinesiology and Anatomy* is the addition of a chapter on the circulatory system. A second significant change is the inclusion of functional task activity analysis in many of the chapters. There are additional photographs to assist students in finding and palpating various muscles and landmarks. The three parts of each chapter remain the same: worksheets to be completed prior to lab to familiarize the student with lab content; lab activities to be completed during lab to clarify understanding and develop palpation skills; and post-lab questions that provide a review.

The layout of this lab manual is similar to that of the second edition and follows closely the layout of Lippert's *Clinical Kinesiology and Anatomy*, fifth edition. The first eight chapters are devoted to basic information that is then applied in the next twelve chapters, which are dedicated to specific body segments. The last two chapters cover posture and gait and the application of information learned in the previous chapters.

The photographs aim to show hand placement for palpation of bones, landmarks, and muscles. On occasion, we altered the position of the subject or the person doing the palpation to obtain an unobstructed view. We once again chose subjects who represent average individuals (not bodybuilders) who more closely resemble the people on whom students likely will be practicing.

LSL
MADM

■ ■ ■ Preface to the Second Edition

This edition of the *Laboratory Manual for Clinical Kinesiology and Anatomy* has several major changes. The addition of several new chapters makes for a closer correlation to *Clinical Kinesiology and Anatomy*, fourth edition, by Lynn Lippert. Photographs showing hand placement for many palpations are another major change. Each chapter still has three parts: worksheets to be completed prior to class, lab activities to be completed in class, and post-lab questions to be completed after class. We believe that students who complete the worksheets prior to class will be familiar with the content and thus prepared to participate during class. The post-lab questions provide the student with the opportunity to review the material after class. Although each chapter directs student learning, each chapter is designed to promote active learning. We believe that students who are actively engaged in their learning are more likely to gain understanding and retain what they have learned.

The first seven chapters are devoted to basic information that is then applied in the next twelve chapters dedicated to specific body segments. The final two chapters are devoted to posture and gait. Examining posture provides students with the opportunity to consider the interrelationships of the various body segments. Walking is our preferred method of mobility when performing our activities of daily living. Having an appreciation for the complexity of walking is necessary to be able to examine someone's gait for effectiveness and efficiency.

A note about the photographs is in order. We attempted to show hand placement, bony landmarks, and muscles in the photographs. To do this, the position of the subject and person performing the palpations may have been altered from the desired position to obtain an unobstructed view. Muscles are not always obvious. Rather than using bodybuilders, we chose subjects who represent average individuals who more closely resemble what students are likely to find when observing their partners.

■ ■ ■ Preface to the First Edition

This laboratory manual is designed to complement Lippert's *Clinical Kinesiology for Physical Therapist Assistants*, but it can be used with other textbooks as well. Each chapter of the manual is divided into three parts: worksheets, lab activities, and post-lab questions.

- The worksheets are designed to assist the student in preparing for the lab session and should be completed by the student prior to class.
- The lab activities are designed to be completed in small groups as part of the lab session. The resources needed for the activities are those readily available and are not costly.
- The post-lab questions are to be completed outside the lab sessions as a review.

We attempted to include the same key concepts in each chapter, as applicable, to allow the students to apply those concepts to a new body region.

The focus of the manual is on understanding normal kinesiology, and thus a selection of normal activities has been presented. We believe that students need to understand normal function before they can appreciate the abnormal. For this reason, the chapters on gait and posture, for example, include a general overview of the normal.

Arthrokinetic concepts involving the convex-concave law are included to provide an introduction to basic joint movements. However, by including this material, we do not mean to imply, suggest, or promote the idea that joint mobilization is an entry-level skill for physical therapist assistants. The concepts of open-chain versus closed-chain activities, having gained popularity in the last few years, has also been included.

This manual is the result of many years of teaching kinesiology to PTA, OTA, and PT students. The authors test-piloted this version during development with the classes they were teaching. Student participation in lab sessions improved, feedback was positive, and suggestions were incorporated into the final version. We thank our students for their patience and their helpful suggestions.

MADM
LSL

ACKNOWLDEDGMENTS

Again, it has been a pleasure to work with Mary Alice Minor. Through all three editions, her eagle eye has seen things I have missed. I am not sure how she finds time in an extremely busy schedule for "one more thing," but I am glad she did. Sal Jepson can never be thanked enough for her wisdom, input, and support. Her original illustrations remain the backbone of this lab manual.

LSL

Lynn Lippert was amazing at keeping us organized even while working on the textbook and climbing mountains to raise money to fight the dread disease of cancer. Scott and Sarah have provided me the support and time away from them to do this third edition. I offer special thanks to Sarah, our photographer. Her professionalism and ability to take charge of her role (even while working with her mother) resulted in an efficient and productive photo shoot and postsession production.

MADM

We thank the people at F. A. Davis for their continued support of this lab manual. We especially thank Melissa Duffield, Acquisitions Editor, who worked so diligently with us. Karen Williams, Developmental Editor, needs a special thanks, as her constructive suggestions for change, attention to detail, and general pleasantness has taken much of the drudgery out of bringing this edition to completion.

Debbie VanDover, PT, MEd; Erin Janssens; and Garon Vasquez were invaluable for their participation and assistance during the photo shoot while Sarah Minor applied her photographic eye and skills. All of their efforts made the photo shoot day successful and enjoyable.

We also wish to congratulate Erin Janssens on her recent appointment as Fire Marshal for the city of Portland, Oregon. She is the first, and highest-ranking, woman to head a division within Portland Fire and Rescue.

LSL & MADM

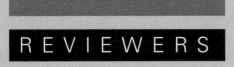

REVIEWERS

Denise Abrams, PT, DPT, MA
Chairperson/Professor
Physical Therapist Assistant
    Program
Broome Community College
Binghamton, New York

Catherine Finch, PT
Instructor
Physical Therapist Assistant Program
Kirkwood Community College
Cedar Rapids, Iowa

Christopher O'Brien, MS, ATC
Clinical Assistant Professor
Athletic Training Education Program
Stony Brook University
Stony Brook, New York

Doreen Olson, MS, OTR
Program Head
Occupational Therapy Assistant
    Program
Western Technical College
La Crosse, Wisconsin

Jill M. Wakabayashi, PTA, MPH
Director
Physical Therapist Assistant Program
Kapi'olani Community College
Honolulu, Hawaii

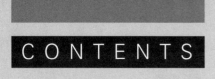

CONTENTS

Basic Clinical Kinesiology
and Anatomy

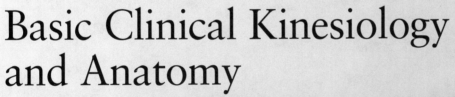

Basic Information

■ ■ ■ Pre-Lab Worksheets

Student's Name _____

Date Due _____

Complete the following questions prior to the lab class.

1. Define:

   Kinesiology:

   _____

   Biomechanics:

   _____

   Kinetics:

   _____

   Kinematics:

   _____

2. The basic information needed to determine the function of a muscle includes:

   _____

   _____

   _____

   _____

3. Fill in the following table by:

   A. Listing characteristics that can be observed while examining a person

   B. Identifying which sensory modality is used to perceive the characteristic

Characteristics	Sensory Modality
Example: Foot slap while walking	Auditory and visual

4. Label Figures 1-1 and 1-2 as either anatomical position or fundamental position.

   Figure 1-1 _____

   Figure 1-2 _____

5. When viewing Figure 1-1, you are observing the person's (anterior/ventral or posterior/dorsal) surface.

   _____

6. When considered together, the right arm and leg can be referred to as (contralateral or ipsilateral).

   _____

7. Using Figure 1-1 and the descriptive terms listed below, describe the location of the following body segments. Terms may be used more than once.

   Medial   Superior   Proximal   Superficial   Anterior
   Lateral   Inferior   Distal   Deep   Posterior

   A. Tibia: The _____ bone of the lower leg

   B. Fibula: The _____ bone of the lower leg

   C. Ribs in relationship to the scapula: _____

D. The elbow joint is at which end of the humerus? _____

E. The brachialis muscle lies underneath the biceps; therefore, it is _____ to the biceps.

F. The head is _____ to the chest.

G. The _____ end of the tibia is at the knee joint.

H. The great toe is on the _____ side of the foot.

I. The eyes are _____ and _____ to the mouth.

J. The radius is on the _____ side of the forearm.

K. The ulna is on the _____ side of the forearm.

L. The scapula is on the _____ side of the trunk.

M. The shoulder girdle is _____ to the pelvic girdle.

N. Skin is _____ to muscle.

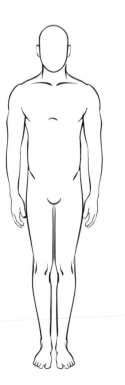

FIGURE 1-1

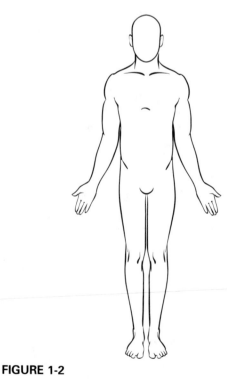

FIGURE 1-2

8. Match the major bone or feature of the body segment with the descriptive term for that segment.

_____ Arm	A. Cervical vertebrae
_____ Forearm	B. Chest
_____ Hand	C. Pelvis
_____ Thigh	D. Radius
_____ Leg	E. Femur
_____ Foot	F. Fingers
_____ Thorax	G. Tibia
_____ Abdomen	H. Humerus
_____ Neck	I. Toes

9. Name and describe the two types of linear motion, which is also called *translatory motion*.

_____

_____

10. In which type of motion do all the parts move:

    A. The same distance: _____

    B. Different distances: _____

11. In Figure 1-3, identify linear motion and angular motion.

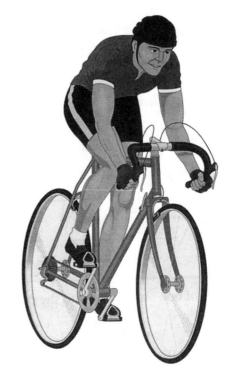

FIGURE 1-3 Bicycle rider.

12. Match the following joint motion with the correct description. The reference position is the anatomical position unless otherwise indicated. Use each answer only once.

_____ Pulling your scapulae together   A. Flexion

_____ Moving your leg toward the midline   B. Extension

_____ Rolling your arm outward   C. Hyperextension

_____ Moving your hand toward the thumb side   D. Abduction

_____ Turning your foot inward   E. Adduction

_____ Moving through a cone-shaped arc   F. Supination

_____ Moving your arm across the body at shoulder level   G. Pronation

_____ Moving your hand down the side of your leg   H. Ulnar deviation

_____ Shoulder motion during bowling backswing   I. Radial deviation

_____ Turning your palm posteriorly   J. Inversion

_____ Moving your arm out to the side   K. Eversion

_____ The position of the knee in standing   L. Lateral rotation

_____ The position of the forearm in anatomical position   M. Medial rotation

_____ Moving the thigh forward and upward   N. Lateral bending

_____ Synonymous with wrist adduction   O. Circumduction

_____ Moving your arm outward from 90 degrees shoulder abduction   P. Horizontal abduction

_____ Moving your foot outward   Q. Horizontal adduction

_____ Moving your scapulae away from the midline   R. Protraction

_____ Turning your arm inward   S. Retraction

■ ■ ■ Lab Activities

Student's Name _____

Date Due _____

1. In a group, students perform the following active motions.

Shoulder:	Flexion	Extension
	Abduction	Abduction
	Horizontal abduction	Horizontal adduction
	Lateral rotation	Medial rotation
Elbow:	Flexion	Extension
Hip:	Flexion	Extension
	Abduction	Adduction
	Lateral rotation	Medial rotation
Knee:	Flexion	Extension

2. Perform the following activities as small groups. Make note of the speed and distance traveled by each person.

   A. Line students up shoulder to shoulder and instruct them to walk across the room keeping their line straight.

   B. Line students up shoulder to shoulder in the middle of the room and instruct them to walk in a circle with the student on the right end as the pivot or anchor.

   C. Repeat activity B with the student on the left end as the pivot or anchor.

   D. Compare the speed of movement of each student in activities A, B, and C.

   _____

   _____

   E. Compare distance traveled by each student in activities A, B, and C.

   _____

   _____

   F. What type of motion is performed in activity A?

   _____

   _____

G. What type of motion is performed in activities B and C?

   _____

   _____

3. To practice palpation, use the finger pads of your right index and middle fingers. Place your fingertips lightly on the anterior surface of your left forearm just proximal to the wrist with your left wrist flexed. Extend your left wrist and note the changing sensations in your fingertips as wrist extension causes the tendons of the wrist and finger flexors to become taut. Move your fingertips medially and laterally (side to side) over the wrist and finger flexor tendons, making note of the changing sensations as you move over the tendons. Note how lightly you are touching and if you are able to palpate the changes. Describe what you feel in your right fingers as you palpated.

   _____

   _____

4. Palpate using your finger pads over the muscles on the lateral aspect of your forearm just distal to the elbow joint. Using light pressure, move your fingers over the area. Describe what you feel (hard, soft, firm).

   _____

   _____

5. With your finger pads over the muscles on the lateral aspect of your forearm just distal to the elbow joint, gradually increase the pressure of your palpation until it becomes slightly uncomfortable. Note how much pressure you are using. Patients, particularly those in pain or with fragile tissues, may not tolerate that amount of pressure. Repeat the muscle palpation using your fingertips. What problem may you encounter palpating with your fingertips?

   _____

   _____

6. Using your finger pads, palpate over the dorsal aspect of the elbow. This is a bony area. Describe what you feel.

   _____

   _____

7. Compare the pressure used to palpate at the wrist, forearm, and elbow. Compare and contrast the sensations you feel at each area.

_____

_____

8. Repeat the previous palpations on your partner. Did you feel the same characteristics as when you palpated yourself? Were you able to adjust your pressure to a comfortable level for your partner while still being able to make the observations you needed?

_____

_____

9. Place the dorsum (back) of your hand on the anterior surface of your partner's foot. Gradually move your hand proximally to just proximal to the knee joint. Describe the temperature of your partner's lower extremity.

_____

_____

10. Practice the following observation and palpation skills on at least two partners.

A. Palpate the biceps brachii muscle belly and tendons. The biceps brachii is on the anterior surface of the humerus. Palpate the relaxed muscle, and then palpate while your partner is contracting the muscle.

1) Describe how you used your hands to palpate (e.g., fingertips, light pressure).

_____

_____

2) Describe the difference you felt when you palpated the relaxed muscle and the contracted muscle. Did what you palpate feel any different when the biceps muscle was contracting?

_____

_____

3) Did contracting the muscle help you to find the tendon?

_____

_____

B. Palpate the medial and lateral epicondyles of the humerus—bony projections on the medial and lateral sides at the elbow.

1) Describe how you used your hands to palpate.

_____

_____

2) Describe what you felt.

_____

_____

C. Palpate the patellar tendon—first with the quadriceps muscle relaxed, and then with your partner contracting the muscle. The patellar tendon is on the anterior proximal tibia just distal to the patella (kneecap).

1) Describe how you used your hands to palpate.

_____

_____

2) Describe what you felt.

_____

_____

3) Did the tendon feel any different when the quadriceps muscle was contracting?

_____

_____

4) If you felt a difference in the tendon between the relaxed state and the contracted state, describe the difference.

_____

_____

5) Did contracting the muscle help you to find the tendon?

———————————————————

———————————————————

D. Palpate your partner's pulse at the radial artery, which is located on the anterior surface of the forearm on the lateral side.

1) Describe how you used your hands to palpate.

———————————————————

———————————————————

2) Describe how the pulse felt (weak, strong, regular, irregular).

———————————————————

———————————————————

E. Palpate the ulnar nerve on the posterior medial aspect of the elbow as the nerve passes just lateral to the medial epicondyle.

1) Describe how you used your hands to palpate the nerve.

———————————————————

———————————————————

2) Describe what you felt.

———————————————————

———————————————————

3) Describe how your partner reacted when you palpated the ulnar nerve with increasing pressure.

———————————————————

———————————————————

11. Posture examination is a visual observation that compares a person's posture to the normal or ideal posture. Symmetry and deviation from normal posture are noted. Because you have not studied posture yet, compare the second of the following two postures to the first, making note of major

changes. Example: In the preferred standing position, your partner shifts a major portion of body weight to the left leg.

A. Observe your partner while he or she is standing erect with weight distributed equally on both feet, which are placed approximately 4 inches apart with the toes pointed forward.

B. Observe your partner standing in his or her preferred standing posture.

C. Describe any major differences between the two postures.

———————————————————

———————————————————

12. To practice visual observation, look at your partner.

A. Describe your partner's physical characteristics such as gender, height, and hair and eye color.

———————————————————

———————————————————

B. Make faces to represent different emotional and physical states such as happy, sad, mad, and in pain. Your partner is to guess which state you are displaying.

13. To practice auditory observations, start with your back to your partner so you cannot see what he or she is doing.

A. While your partner is facing away from you, perform some ADLs such as taking off your shoes, removing your shirt, and walking. Ask your partner to describe what they heard and to tell you what activity you performed.

———————————————————

———————————————————

B. If you know how, take your partner's blood pressure, paying particular attention to the sounds rather than the pressure reading. What sounds did you hear? Were there periods of silence? If so, when?

———————————————————

———————————————————

C. Using a stethoscope, listen to your partner's heart and lungs. Describe the sounds you heard.

_____

14. Perform as many of the following motions as possible while standing, sitting, lying supine, and side-lying.

Shoulder girdle: Elevation and depression
Protraction and retraction
Upward and downward rotation

Shoulder: Flexion, extension, and
hyperextension
Abduction and adduction
Horizontal abduction and
adduction
Medial and lateral rotation
Circumduction

Elbow: Flexion and extension

Forearm: Supination and pronation

Wrist: Flexion and extension
Radial and ulnar deviation
Circumduction

Finger: Flexion and extension
Abduction and adduction

Thumb: Flexion and extension
Abduction and adduction
Opposition

Hip: Flexion, extension, and
hyperextension
Abduction and adduction
Medial and lateral rotation
Circumduction

Knee: Flexion and extension

Ankle: Dorsiflexion and plantar flexion
Inversion and eversion

Toe: Extension and flexion

15. Perform the previously listed movements in random order and have your partner name the movement that you are performing.

■ ■ ■ Post-Lab Questions

Student's Name _____

Date Due _____

After you have completed the Worksheets and Lab Activities, answer the following questions without using your book or notes. When finished, check your answers.

1. List the senses used when observing a person.

   _____

   _____

2. List at least two structures of the body on the:

   A. Anterior surface:

   _____

   _____

   B. Lateral surface:

   _____

   _____

   C. Posterior surface:

   _____

   _____

3. Define the following terms:

   A. Kinesiology:

   _____

   B. Flexion:

   _____

   _____

   C. Medial rotation:

   _____

   D. Osteokinematics:

   _____

4. List at least two structures of the body that are:

   A. Superior to the waist:

   _____

   _____

   B. Lateral to the sternum:

   _____

   _____

   C. Inferior to the hip:

   _____

   _____

   D. Distal to the elbow:

   _____

   _____

5. What type of motion is occurring in the following activities?

Activity	Type of Motion
Knee flexion	
Bowling ball rolling down the gutter	
Rounding the curve when running on a track	
A somersault	
A curve ball in baseball	

Skeletal System

■ ■ ■ Pre-Lab Worksheets

Student's Name _____

Date Due _____

Complete the following questions prior to the lab class.

1. List five functions of the skeletal system:

   _____

   _____

   _____

   _____

   _____

2. Complete the following table, indicating whether the listed body parts are part of the axial or appendicular skeleton.

Body Part	Axial	Appendicular
Arms		
Head		
Vertebrae		
Lower extremity		

3. Describe compact bone:

   _____

   _____

4. Describe cancellous bone:

   _____

   _____

5. Bone is made up of [how much] _____ organic material and _____ inorganic material.

6. Where are osteoclasts located?

   _____

7. On Figure 2-1, label the parts of a long bone, using the terms listed below:

Epiphysis	Diaphysis
Endosteum	Periosteum
Epiphyseal plate	Medullary canal
Metaphysis	

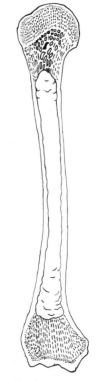

FIGURE 2-1 Longitudinal cross section of a long bone.

8. Which of the following is located at the ends of long bones?

   A._____ Pressure epiphysis

   B. _____ Traction epiphysis

9. What covers most of a bone's surface, and what is its purpose?

   _____

10. Where does longitudinal bone growth occur?

   _____

11. Complete the following table, indicating whether the terms are related to compact or cancellous bone.

Characteristic	Compact Bone	Cancellous Bone
Porous and spongy		
Hard and dense		
Covers outside of bone		
Inside portion of bone		

12. On Figure 2-2, label the bones, using the terms listed below.

Irregular bone   Long bone   Flat bone   Short bone

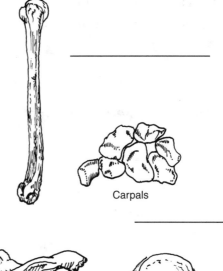

Carpals

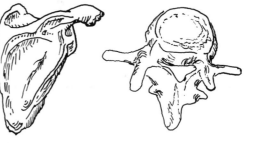

FIGURE 2-2 Types of bones.

■ ■ ■ Lab Activities

Student's Name _____

Date Due _____

1. The patella can be considered a sesamoid bone. With your partner long sitting (sitting on a mat or table with knees extended) and with muscles relaxed, grasp the patella with the thumb and index finger of one hand proximally and the thumb and index finger of the other hand distally.
   - Gently move the patella medially and laterally, superiorly and inferiorly. Note the amount of motion in each direction.
   - Palpate for other sesamoid bones such as on either side of the flexor hallucis longus on the bottom of the foot, at the head of the first metatarsal, and the flexor tendons of the thumb near the metacarpophalangeal and interphalangeal joints.

2. On your partner, palpate the following markings, and describe where on what bone that marking was found.

Marking	Location
Crest	
Epicondyle	
Tuberosity	

3. Using skeletons and models, find examples of the following bony landmarks. Describe where the landmark is located (using terms such as *proximal/distal, medial/lateral, superior/inferior,* and *anterior/posterior*) and give the name of the bone where you found the landmark.

Landmark	Location
Example: Trochanter	Proximal and lateral on femur
Foramen	
Fossa	
Groove	
Meatus	

Sinus	
Condyle	
Eminence	
Facet	
Head	
Crest	
Epicondyle	
Line	
Spine	
Tubercle	
Tuberosity	
Trochanter	

4. On a skeleton, identify the bones and bone groups that make up the axial skeleton and the appendicular skeleton. List the bones that are found in each group.

Skeleton	Bones and Bone Groups (e.g., carpals, ribs)
Axial	
Appendicular	

5. Using bones in the bone box, arrange the bones of the upper extremity and the bones of the lower extremity in proper anatomical orientation to one another to create the appendicular skeleton. Arrange an entire right side or left side.

6. Examine a mid-shaft cross section of a long bone and describe the type and appearance of the bone.

_____

_____

7. Examine a cross section of the epiphysis of a long bone:

   A. Describe the type and appearance of the bone.

   _____

   _____

   B. Name the type of bone.

   _____

   _____

   C. What type of bone comprises the outer layer of bone?

   _____

   _____

8. Using disarticulated bones, identify the structures listed below on several different bones. Can all the parts be found on each bone? _____

   Epiphysis   Epiphyseal plate   Diaphysis
   Endosteum   Metaphysis   Periosteum

9. Using the skeleton and models:

   A. Find examples of the following types of bones.

   B. Name an example of each type of bone.

Type of Bone	Example
Short	
Flat	
Long	
Irregular	
Sesamoid	

■ ■ ■ Post-Lab Questions

Student's Name _____

Date Due _____

After you have completed the worksheets and lab activities, answer the following questions without using your book or notes. When finished, check your answers.

1. The function of the skull is to protect the brain. What is a disadvantage of the mature skull?

   _____

2. Describe the function of the:

   A. Axial skeleton:

   _____

   _____

   B. Appendicular skeleton:

   _____

   _____

3. What is the result of a loss of the inorganic component of bone?

   _____

   _____

4. Why is cancellous bone lighter than compact bone?

   _____

   _____

5. How does a traction epiphysis affect the shape of a bone?

   _____

6. What is the function of the following parts of a bone?

Bone Part	Function
Epiphysis	
Epiphyseal plate	
Diaphysis	
Medullary canal	
Endosteum	
Osteoclasts	
Metaphysis	
Periosteum	

7. Identify whether the types of bones listed below are typically part of the axial or appendicular skeleton.

Type of Bone	Axial Skeleton	Appendicular Skeleton
Long		
Short		
Flat		
Irregular		

8. Match the following descriptions of bone markings with the correct term. Use each term only once.

_____ Projection above a condyle   A. Sinus

_____ Rounded projection at the end of a joint   B. Tubercle

_____ Hole   C. Crest

_____ Spongelike space filled with air   D. Spine

_____ Tube-shaped opening   E. Foramen

_____ Rounded projection beyond a narrow neck portion   F. Condyle

_____ Less prominent ridge   G. Groove

_____ Large, rounded projection   H. Fossa

_____ Flat articular surface   I. Tuberosity

_____ Very large projection   J. Head

_____ Large depression   K. Meatus

_____ Linear depression   L. Trochanter

_____ Ridge   M. Epicondyle

_____ Small, rounded projection   N. Line

_____ Sharp projection   O. Facet

9. Where does growth of long bones occur?

_____

10. What contributes to the development of bony projections and processes such as tubercles and tuberosities?

_____

_____

11. What function do sesamoid bones serve?

_____

_____

Articular System

■ ■ ■ Pre-Lab Worksheets

Student's Name _____

Date Due _____

Complete the following questions prior to the lab class.

1. What are the three basic types of joints?

   A. _____

   B. _____

   C. _____

2. Which type of joint is the most typical of the joints of the appendicular skeleton?

   _____

3. Rank the three basic types of joints from most to least amount of movement permitted.

   Most: _____

   _____

   Least: _____

4. Match the type of fibrous joint with the appropriate description.

   _____ Synarthrosis   A. Bolted together

   _____ Syndesmosis   B. Ligaments join the bones

   _____ Gomphosis   C. Fibrous periosteum between bones

5. Give an example of each of the following types of fibrous joints.

   A. Synarthrosis: _____

   B. Syndesmosis: _____

   C. Gomphosis: _____

6. What is another name for a synovial joint?

   _____

7. Which of the three basic types of joints provides for:

   A. Mobility: _____

   B. Stability: _____

8. List an example of each of the following synovial joints:

   A. Nonaxial joint: _____

   B. Uniaxial joint: _____

   C. Biaxial joint: _____

   D. Triaxial joint: _____

9. Label the drawing of a synovial joint using the following terms (Fig. 3-1):

   Ligament   Joint space   Synovial membrane   Joint capsule

   Bone   Synovial fluid   Articular cartilage

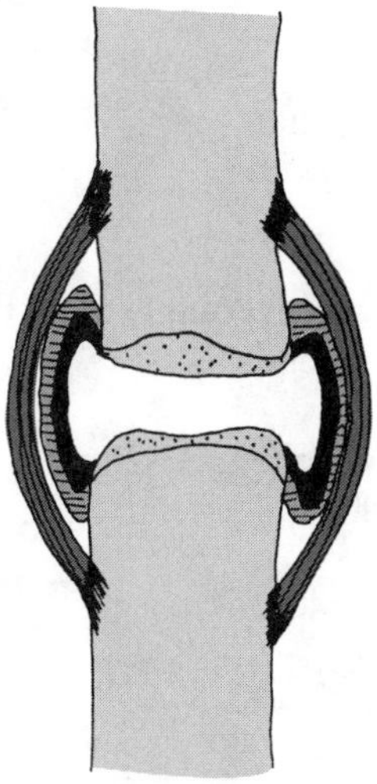

FIGURE 3-1 Synovial joint.

10. Match the following descriptions of parts of a synovial joint with the correct term. Use each term only once.

_____ Enclosed cavity filled with fluid that prevents friction on moving parts   A. Joint capsule

_____ Strong cord of connective tissue that attaches a muscle to another part   B. Synovial membrane

_____ The inside lining of the joint capsule   C. Synovial fluid

_____ Strong, fibrous connective tissue band that attaches bone to bone   D. Tendon

_____ Flat, thin, fibrous sheet of connective tissue that attaches a muscle to another part   E. Articular cartilage

_____ Fibrous connective tissue that surrounds a joint   F. Bursa

_____ Sheath of connective tissue that surrounds a muscle   G. Aponeurosis

_____ Fluid secreted from inside the lining of the joint capsule that lubricates the joint   H. Ligament

_____ Smooth covering of bone ends   I. Fascia

11. For each drawing (Figs. 3-2 through 3-4), fill in the blanks regarding planes and axes.

    A. In Figure 3-2:

    This is the _____ plane. It is associated with the _____ axis.

Describe the direction of the axis:

_____

List the motions that occur in this plane around this axis:

_____

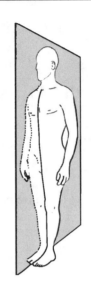

FIGURE 3-2

    B. In Figure 3-3:

    This is the _____ plane. It is associated with the _____ axis.

    Describe the direction of the axis:

_____

    List the motions that occur in this plane around this axis:

_____

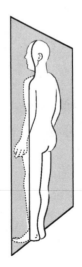

FIGURE 3-3

C. In Figure 3-4:

This is the _____ plane. It is associated with the _____ axis.

Describe the direction of the axis:

_____

List the motions that occur in this plane around this axis:

_____

12. For each of the following joints, indicate the degrees of freedom for that joint.

Joint	One	Two	Three
Shoulder			
Elbow			
Wrist			
Hip			
Knee			
Ankle			

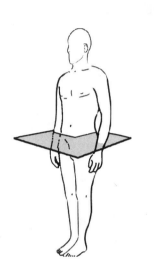

FIGURE 3-4

■ ■ ■ Lab Activities

Student's Name _____

Date Due _____

1. In a group, students perform the following motions as active motions.

Shoulder girdle	Elevation Protraction	Depression Retraction
Shoulder	Flexion	Extension Hyperextension
	Abduction	Adduction
	Horizontal abduction	Horizontal adduction
	Medial rotation	Lateral rotation
Elbow	Flexion	Extension
Forearm	Supination	Pronation
Wrist	Flexion	Extension
	Radial deviation	Ulnar deviation
Thumb	Flexion	Extension
	Abduction	Opposition
Hip	Flexion	Extension Hyperextension
	Abduction	Adduction
	Medial rotation	Lateral rotation
Knee	Flexion	Extension
	Medial rotation	Lateral rotation
Ankle	Dorsiflexion	Plantarflexion
Foot	Inversion	Eversion

2. Using models, locate the components of synovial joints listed below, and note the relationship of the components to one another.

Bones	Ligaments	Capsule
Hyaline cartilage	Articular cartilage	Synovial membrane
Menisci	Labrum	Disks

3. Using a skeleton, identify and examine examples of the following types of joints:

A. Fibrous joints:

Synarthrosis: _____

Syndesmosis: _____

Gomphosis: _____

B. Cartilaginous joints (also named *amphiarthrodial joints*) _____

C. Synovial joints (also named *diarthrodial joints*)

_____

D. Nonaxial joints _____

E. Uniaxial joints _____

F. Biaxial joints (also referred to as *condyloid joints*) _____

G. Triaxial joints (also referred to as *ball and socket joints*)

_____

4. Standing next to a wall so that your left shoulder and hip are against the wall, perform flexion and extension of each of the following left extremity joints individually: shoulder, elbow, hip, and knee.

A. In what plane were you moving?

_____

B. What is the axis for that plane?

_____

5. Standing in anatomical position with your back against a wall, perform the following motions:
   - Slide one arm along the wall until your hand points toward the ceiling.
   - Return your arm to anatomical position by moving it along the wall.
   - Move one leg to the side, sliding your heel along the wall.
   - Return your leg to anatomical position, keeping it in contact with the wall.

   A. What motion did you perform as you moved your extremity away from your body?

   _____

   B. What motion did you perform as you moved your extremity back to the anatomical position?

   _____

   C. In what plane were you moving?

   _____

   D. What is the axis for that plane?

   _____

6. Standing facing a counter with your upper arm close to your body, your elbow at 90 degrees of flexion, and your forearm pronated, place your hand palm down on the countertop. Keeping your hand in contact with the surface of the countertop, move your palm:
   - away from the midline of your body.
   - toward the midline of your body.

   A. What motion did you perform when your palm moved away from the midline of your body?

   _____

   B. What motion did you perform when your palm moved toward the midline of your body?

   _____

   C. In what plane were you moving?

   _____

   D. What is the axis for that plane?

   _____

7. Sitting on a chair, move your lower leg:
   - away from the midline of your body.
   - toward the midline of your body.

   A. What motion did you perform when you moved your leg away from the midline of your body?

   _____

   B. What motion did you perform when you moved your leg toward the midline of your body?

   _____

   C. In what plane were you moving?

   _____

   D. What is the axis for that plane?

   _____

8. Using models of joints, a skeleton, and your own body, move the joints listed below through the motions normally permitted to determine the degrees of freedom and the specific motions. Record your findings on the following chart.

Joint	Degrees of Freedom	Motions
Shoulder		
Elbow		
Wrist		
Hip		
Knee		

9. What is the relationship between the degrees of freedom and the types of joint?

   _____

10. Compare models of the acetabulum and glenoid fossa with and without their labrum. How does the presence or absence of the labrum change the structure of the joint?

   _____

   _____

■ ■ ■ Post-Lab Questions

Student's Name _____

Date Due _____

After you have completed the worksheets and lab activities, answer the following questions without using your book or notes. When finished, check your answers.

1. Compare and contrast fibrous joints, cartilaginous joints, and synovial joints.

   A. What are the structural similarities?

   _____

   _____

   _____

   B. What is the difference in the amount of motion permitted?

   _____

   _____

2. Diarthrodial joints can be classified based on their characteristics. Fill in the blanks with the appropriate information. There may be more than one example.

Number of Axes	Shape of Joint	Joint Motions Allowed	Example

3. What structure(s) may reinforce a joint capsule?

   _____

4. List the structure(s) that lubricate and supply nutrition to joint surfaces.

   _____

5. List the five features of a synovial joint.

   _____

   _____

   _____

6. Place a check in the box that corresponds to the motions that generally occur in each plane about its axis:

Planes/ Axes	Flexion/ Extension	Adduction/ Abduction	Medial/ Lateral Rotation
Sagittal plane/ Frontal axis			
Frontal plane/ Sagittal axis			
Transverse plane/ Vertical axis			

7. For the joints listed, indicate in which plane the joint normally can actively move.

Plane	Shoulder	Wrist	Knee	Ankle
Sagittal				
Frontal				
Transverse				

8. Define degrees of freedom.

   _____

9. Give examples of joints that have:

   A. One degree of freedom: _____

   B. Two degrees of freedom: _____

   C. Three degrees of freedom: _____

10. Generally the joints of which of the following have more degrees of freedom?

   _____ Axial skeleton _____ Appendicular skeleton

11. The more degrees of freedom a joint has, the more likely its function is

   _____ mobility. _____ stability.

12. Underline the correct term inside the parentheses:

   The axial skeleton functions to provide (mobility/stability) for the (mobility/stability) of the appendicular skeleton. The abilities of the axial and appendicular skeleton combine to permit the myriad of movements the human uses in daily activities.

Arthrokinematics

■ ■ ■ Pre-Lab Worksheets

Student's Name _____

Date Due _____

Complete the following questions prior to the lab class.

1. Match the types of normal end feels with their definitions.

   _____ Soft, with considerable give   A. Bony end feel

   _____ Hard and abrupt limit   B. Soft tissue stretch

   _____ Firm, with slight give   C. Soft tissue approximation

2. Match the types of abnormal end feels with their definitions.

   _____ Soft, "wet sponge" feel   A. Bony

   _____ Rebound movement at end of ROM   B. Boggy

   _____ Sudden hard stop before end of ROM   C. Muscle spasm

   _____ Reflex muscle guarding   D. Empty

   _____ Pain, not mechanical constraint, limits movement   E. Springy block

3. Match the following terms with their definitions.

   _____ Passive oscillatory motions applied by external force   A. Component movements

   _____ Forceful external force applied within a short range   B. Joint play

   _____ Accessory joint movements resulting from external force   C. Joint mobilization

   _____ Motions that facilitate active motion   D. Manipulation

4. A convex surface is curved _____.

5. A concave surface is curved _____.

6. An ovoid joint is formed by two bones forming a _____ relationship. One bone's surface is _____, and the other is _____.

7. Each of the two bones that make a sellar or saddle-shaped joint have a joint surface that is _____ and a joint surface that is _____.

8. Match the terms for arthrokinematic motion with their definitions.

   _____ Same point on each surface remains in contact with each other   A. Roll

   _____ One point on a joint surface contacts new points on the other surface   B. Spin

   _____ New points on each surface come into contact throughout the motion   C. Glide

9. Apply the concave-convex rule to identify the type of joint surface (concave/convex) moving in each of the following statements.

   A. Which type of joint surface moves in the opposite direction as the moving body segment?

   _____

   B. Which type of joint surface moves in the same direction as the moving body segment moves?

   _____

10. Match the joint surface position with its description.

   _____ Close-packed position   A. Congruent joint surfaces

   _____ Open-packed position   B. Incongruent joint surfaces

11. Match the type of force with its definition.

   _____ Joint surfaces are pulled apart   A. Traction, distraction, or tension force

   _____ Joint surfaces move parallel and in opposite directions of each other   B. Approximation, compression force

   _____ Joint surfaces are pushed closer together   C. Shear force

12. When bending the trunk to the right:

   A. The force acting on the right side is _____ because the curve on the right side is _____.

   B. The force acting on the left side is _____ because the curve on the left side is _____.

■ ■ ■ Lab Activities

Student's Name _____

Date Due _____

1. Passively extend your partner's elbow. When you reach the end of the range, the end feel is hard. This is because the humerus and ulna come together to lock the elbow in place. The term used to describe this end feel is _____.

2. Have your partner lie supine. Passively flex his or her hip. When you reach the end of the range, the end feel is soft. There is more "give" than at the end of elbow extension. This is because there is much more muscle bulk, and the femur and acetabulum do not lock together. The term used to describe this end feel is _____.

3. With your partner lying prone, passively hyperextend her or his hip. When you reach the end of the range, the end feel is firm. This is because there is tension on the anterior ligaments and muscles of the hip. The term used to describe this end feel is _____.

4. Perform the following on several people. Describe the end feel of each motion.

Motion	End Feel
Elbow flexion	
Elbow extension	
Wrist flexion	
Knee extension	
Hip flexion with knee flexion	
Hip flexion with knee extended	

5. Perform shoulder flexion, first while maintaining medial rotation and then with lateral rotation. Compare the amount of range of motion achieved with each movement.

   A. Which movement has greater ROM?

   _____ Medial rotation _____ Lateral rotation

   B. This is an example of what type of arthrokinematic motion? _____

6. Sitting and facing your partner, with your partner's hand supported on a table, grasp your partner's index finger middle phalange with one hand and her or his index finger distal phalange with your other hand. While holding the middle phalange stable, move the distal phalange from side to side.

   A. Can a person perform this movement voluntarily? _____

   B. What is this movement called?

   _____

7. Using a skeleton and bones, locate bones whose articular surfaces have the following characteristics. Describe where on the bone the characteristic is found (proximal/distal; medial/lateral; anterior/posterior).

   A. Concave surface:

Bone	Location
Scapula	
Radius	
Tibia	
Ilium	
Sacrum	

   B. Convex surface:

Bone	Location
Humerus	
Femur	
Talus	
Sacrum	

8. Examine the carpometacarpal (CMC) joint of the thumb and fingers.

   A. How do the joint surfaces of the thumb differ from the joint surfaces of the fingers?

   _____

   _____

   B. What is the type of joint for each?

   _____

   _____

9. Observe the distal end of a femur and the proximal end of a tibia.

   A. Which has the larger articular surface?

   _____

   B. Move the tibia on the femur as if performing extension and flexion. Does the tibia move over the entire articular surface of the femur?

   _____

   C. As you move the tibia on the femur as if performing extension, move the femur posteriorly on the tibia. Did the tibia move over more of the articular surface of the femur this time?

   _____

   D. The posterior movement of the femur is an example of what kind of arthrokinematic motion?

   _____

10. Using a skeleton or the articulated upper extremity bones, observe the proximal end of the radius while performing pronation and supination.

    A. Describe the movement of the radius on the humerus.

    _____

    B. This movement is an example of what type of arthrokinematic motion?

    _____

11. Using a skeleton or disarticulated upper extremity bones, observe the movement of the head of the humerus while performing shoulder joint medial and lateral rotation. Indicate which of the following movements occurs as the humerus moves on the glenoid fossa.

    _____ Roll _____ Spin _____ Glide

12. Place two small sticky notes with large dots on the lateral surface of your partner's arm, with one dot over the lateral epicondyle at the elbow and the other at the shoulder on the greater tubercle. As your partner slowly flexes the shoulder, observe the positions of the dots.

    A. When performing shoulder flexion, which joint surface is moving—the concave or the convex surface?

    _____

    B. In the starting position, the dot at the elbow is _____ to the dot at the shoulder.

    C. At the end of shoulder flexion, the dot at the elbow is _____ to the dot at the shoulder.

    D. This is an example of the concave-convex rule describing movement of the convex joint surface. According to the concave-convex rule, the convex joint surface moves in the _____ direction as the body segment's motion.

13. Place two small sticky notes with large dots on the lateral aspect of your partner's lower leg, with one dot over the lateral malleolus and the other over the head of the fibula. Observe the positions of the dots as your partner performs knee flexion, moving the tibia on the femur.

    A. When performing knee flexion and extension moving the tibia on the femur, which joint surface is moving—the concave or the convex surface?

    _____

    B. In what direction did the proximal dot move during flexion?

    _____

    C. In what direction did the distal dot move during flexion?

    _____

    D. This is an example of the concave-convex rule describing movement of the concave joint surface. According to the concave-convex rule, the concave joint surface moves in the _____ direction as the body segment's motion.

14. Using a skeleton or bones, observe the close-packed
    or open-packed positions of the following joints.

Joint	Close-Packed	Open-Packed
Glenohumeral	Abduction and lateral rotation	55° abduction, 30° horizontal adduction
Elbow: ulnohumeral	Extension	70° flexion, 10° supination
Interphalangeal	Full extension	Slight flexion
Hip	Full extension and medial rotation	30° flexion, 30° abduction, and slight lateral rotation
Knee	Full extension and lateral rotation of tibia	25° flexion
Ankle: talocrural	Full dorsiflexion	10° plantar flexion, midway between inversion and eversion

■ ■ ■ ■ Post-Lab Questions

Student's Name _____

Date Due _____

After you have completed the worksheets and lab activities, answer the following questions without using your book or notes. When finished, check your answers.

1. Give an example of each of the following and identify the structure(s) responsible for the end feel. Try to use examples not described in the textbook.

   A. Bony end feel: _____

   B. Soft tissue stretch: _____

   C. Soft tissue approximation: _____

   D. Empty end feel: _____

   E. Springy block: _____

2. What component motion accompanies

   A. shoulder abduction? _____

   B. knee extension? _____

3. A saddle joint is unique because each bone of the joint has surfaces that are

   _____.

4. Give an example of each of the following:

   A. Joint movement with large amount of roll:

   _____

   B. Joint movement with large amount of glide:

   _____

   _____

   C. Joint movement with large amount of spin:

   _____

5. When a person assumes sitting from standing, the knee is flexing.

   A. When performing this movement, is the concave surface moving on the convex surface or is the convex surface moving on the concave surface? Underline the correct response.

   B. Based on this example, according to the concave-convex rule, when the _____ surface moves on the _____ surface rule, the _____ joint surface moves in the _____ direction as the body segment movement.

6. Is accessory motion or joint play possible in a close-packed or an open-packed position? Why?

   _____

   _____

7. When bending to the right, the soft tissue that is being lengthened is on the _____ right side. _____ left side.

8. In the sitting position, turn your head and upper body while keeping your lower body stationary. This movement is _____, and it occurs in the _____ plane about the _____ axis. The force producing this motion is a _____ force.

9. Describe typical exercises or activities that apply

   A. a traction force through the upper extremities.

   _____

   B. an approximation force through the lower extremities.

   _____

10. When bending the trunk to the left:

    A. On which side are structures compressed?

    _____

    B. On which side are structures under tension?

    _____

    C. With the trunk erect, what force is applied to the structures of the trunk as the trunk is twisted to one side or the other?

    _____

11. When you passively hyperextend a person's hip through full range of motion, the end feel is firm. This is because there is tension on the anterior ligaments and muscles of the hip. The term used to describe this is _____.

Muscular System

■ ■ ■ Pre-Lab Worksheets

Student's Name _____

Date Due _____

Complete the following questions prior to the lab class.

1. Match the following terms with their definition.

_____	Muscle contraction without joint movement	A. Reversal of muscle action
_____	Distance between maximum contracted and extended length	B. Normal resting length
_____	The origin of the contracting muscle moves toward the insertion	C. Tone
_____	Constant speed with variable resistance	D. Tenodesis
_____	Not as powerful as the prime mover	E. Isometric contraction
_____	Slight tension in a muscle	F. Isokinetic contraction
_____	Position when muscle is unstimulated	G. Assisting mover
_____	Can produce hand opening and closing	H. Muscle excursion

2. Muscles have origins and insertions. Which is generally proximal?

_____

3. A. The sternocleidomastoid muscle typically flexes the head and neck. The mastoid process (on the head) is the insertion and the sternum and clavicle are the origin. Is the origin moving toward the insertion, or is the insertion moving toward the origin during flexion of the head and neck?

_____

B. When you have worked hard and are short of breath, the sternocleidomastoid helps you to take deeper breathes by lifting the chest. In this case, is the origin moving toward the insertion, or is the insertion moving toward the origin?

_____

C. Muscles acting in this manner are said to be performing a _____.

4. Match the muscle with the characteristic associated with its name.

	Location	Shape	Action	Number of Heads	Attachments	Direction of Fibers	Muscle Size
Rhomboids							
Abductor digiti minimi							
Biceps brachii							
Quadriceps femoris							
Pectoralis major							
Gluteus medius							
Sternocleidomastoid							

5. Using the following terms, identify the muscle shapes illustrated in Figure 5-1.

Triangular   Strap   Rhomboidal   Fusiform
Bipennate   Multipennate   Unipennate

6. Using the terms listed in question 5, name the type of muscle fiber arrangement for each muscle:

Muscle	Fiber Arrangement
Deltoid	
Pectoralis major	
Flexor pollicis longus	
Biceps brachii	
Rectus femoris	
Sternocleidomastoid	
Rhomboids	

FIGURE 5-1 Muscle shapes.

7. Match the muscle characteristic with the correct description. Use each term only once.

_____ Ability to be stretched beyond normal resting length   A. Irritability

_____ Ability to receive and respond to a stimulus   B. Contractility

_____ Ability to produce tension   C. Extensibility

_____ Ability to return to normal length   D. Elasticity

8. A muscle with a resting length of 4 inches can be shortened approximately 2 inches and lengthened 4 inches. Therefore, it has an excursion of _____.

9. A muscle that cannot be lengthened simultaneously over all the joints it crosses is said to be

    _____ actively insufficient.

    _____ passively insufficient.

10. Stretching a multijoint muscle is achieved by positioning the joints to cause the muscle to be in its

    _____ shortened position.

    _____ resting position.

    _____ lengthened position.

    _____ lengthened position at some joints and shortened at other joints.

11. The advantage of a two-joint muscle is that it can maintain greater contractility through its range, because while it is _____ over one joint, it is being _____ over the other joint.

12. Identify the type of muscle contraction described below as eccentric (E) or concentric (C).

    _____ Lengthening contraction

    _____ Shortening contraction

    _____ Insertion moves toward origin

    _____ Insertion moves away from origin

    _____ Isotonic contraction

    _____ Muscle contraction moves the body segment against gravity

    _____ Muscle contraction slows the pull of gravity on the body segment

13. Complete the following statements using the terms listed below:

    Agonist   Antagonist   Cocontraction
    Neutralizer   Stabilizers   Synergists

    A. The shoulder girdle muscles act as _____ when one lifts a book off the table.

    B. When a muscle acts to eliminate undesired motions during an activity, it is functioning as a _____.

C. Contracting the quadriceps and hamstring muscles simultaneously is an example of _____.

D. Muscles that are primarily responsible for producing a specific movement are called the _____.

E. When the biceps are contracting, the triceps muscle is the _____.

F. The elbow has three muscles that can produce flexion. When more than one muscle is working, the muscles are acting as _____.

G. When the wrist flexors and extensors produce ulnar deviation, each muscle is also acting as a _____.

14. The angle of pull of a muscle is determined, in part, by the relationship of the muscle to the _____ it crosses.

15. Indicate whether each of the following activities is an example of an open kinetic chain (O) or a closed kinetic chain (C).

    _____ A. The upper extremity when one is walking and carrying a book bag

    _____ B. The upper extremity when one is doing push-ups

    _____ C. The upper extremity when one is supported on crutches

    _____ D. The lower extremities when one is swinging from an overhead bar

    _____ E. The lower extremities when one is performing wall slides

    _____ F. The lower extremity being used to kick a ball

■ ■ ■ Lab Activities

Student's Name _____

Date Due _____

1. Palpate the origins and insertions of the following muscles. Indicate which, origin or insertion, is located proximally and which is located distally. Remember that the proximal attachment is also usually the more stable attachment, and the distal attachment is more movable.

Muscle	Origin	Insertion	Proximal	Distal
Brachioradialis	Lateral supracondylar ridge on the humerus	Styloid process of the radius		
Teres minor	Axillary border of scapula	Greater tubercle of humerus		
Rectus abdominis	Pubis	Costal cartilages of fifth, sixth, and seventh ribs		
Sartorius	Anterior superior iliac spine	Proximal medial aspect of tibia		
Soleus	Posterior tibia and fibula	Posterior calcaneus		

2. Using pictures from the Lippert text, locate the muscles listed below on your partner and yourself. Use a skin pencil or a water-soluble marker to draw over your partner's muscles, showing the muscle fiber arrangement.

Deltoid   Pectoralis major   Flexor pollicis longus

Biceps brachii   Rectus femoris   Sternocleidomastoid

Rhomboids

3. Have your partner assume a supine position. Standing next to your partner's right lower extremity, place the heel of her or his lower extremity in the palm of your right hand. Place your left hand under your partner's right thigh.

- Slowly flex and then extend your partner's hip and knee simultaneously. Note the amount of "resistance" you feel while moving your partner's lower extremity. Some people have a difficult time letting someone else move their body parts; however, if your partner is relaxed, you will feel the normal resting tone of her or his lower extremity muscles.

4. With your partner in a supine position, stand next to her or his right lower extremity and place the heel of her or his lower extremity in the palm of your right hand. Place your left hand under your partner's right thigh.

- Slowly flex and then extend your partner's hip and knee simultaneously. Note the amount of hip flexion.
- Next, slowly flex and then extend your partner's hip while keeping the knee extended (straight). Note the amount of hip flexion your partner has when the knee remains extended. Hip flexion with the knee extended (straight) is known as a straight leg raise—SLR.

A. Was the amount of hip flexion more, the same, or less with knee extended compared to hip flexion with the knee flexed? _____

B. Was the result what you expected? _____

C. Is this an example of active or passive insufficiency? _____

D. Which muscle(s) was (were) being lengthened simultaneously over all the joints they crossed when you moved your partner through the SLR?

_____

_____

5. Perform the following activities on your partner:
   - With your partner in a supine position, perform simultaneous hip and knee flexion. Note the amount of knee flexion obtained when the hip is flexed.
   - Have your partner assume a prone position. Align the thigh in anatomical position. Slowly flex the knee of the same lower extremity you had moved when your partner was supine. Note the amount of knee flexion motion present now that the hip is extended.

   A. Was the amount of knee flexion more, the same, or less with the hip extended compared to knee flexion with the hip flexed? _____

   B. Was the result what you expected? _____

   C. Is this an example of active or passive insufficiency? _____

   D. Which muscle(s) was (were) being lengthened simultaneously over all the joints they cross when you moved your partner through knee flexion with the hip extended? _____

6. Perform the following activities on your partner.
   - With your partner sitting over the side of a treatment table with her or his knee at about 90 degrees of flexion, resist your partner's isometric knee flexion. Note how strong the knee flexors are in this position.
   - Have your partner assume a prone position with hip extended and the same knee flexed to 90 degrees. Repeat the resisted isometric contraction of the knee flexors, noting the strength of the knee flexors.
   - Have your partner assume a prone position with hip extended and flex her or his knee through as much of its range of motion as possible (more than 90 degrees). Repeat the resisted isometric contraction at the end of the motion, noting the strength of the knee flexors. Be cautious with the resistance offered, because your partner may develop a muscle cramp.

   A. Describe the hip and knee position in these three scenarios:

Hip and Knee Position	Hip	Knee
Sitting on side of table		
Prone with knee at 90°		
Prone with maximum knee flexion		

B. Was the strength of the knee flexors the same in all three positions? _____

C. If not, in which position were the knee flexors strongest? _____ weakest? _____

D. Is the weakest position an example of active or passive insufficiency? _____

7. When your partner performs the maximum knee flexion possible in the prone position, how do you determine if she or he is experiencing active insufficiency of the knee flexors or passive insufficiency of the knee extensors?

   _____

   _____

   _____

   _____

8. As a general rule, the following statements describe muscle contractions in relation to gravity:

   A. When joint movement occurs against gravity, the agonist performs which type of contraction?

   _____ Isometric _____ Concentric _____ Eccentric _____ None

   B. When joint movement occurs against gravity, the antagonist performs which type of contraction?

   _____ Isometric _____ Concentric _____ Eccentric _____ None

   C. When a joint is moved against gravity by action of another joint, the agonist performs which type of contraction to prevent movement?

   _____ Isometric _____ Concentric _____ Eccentric _____ None

   D. When joint movement occurs in the same direction that gravity would produce movement, the agonist performs which type of contraction?

   _____ Isometric _____ Concentric _____ Eccentric _____ None

   E. When performing an eccentric contraction, the agonist is acting to

   _____ overcome gravity. _____ slow down gravity.

   F. When performing a concentric contraction, the agonist is acting to

   _____ overcome gravity. _____ slow down gravity.

9. Throughout this lab manual, you will be asked to analyze activities to determine the type of muscle contractions required to perform the activity. In the supine position, perform a straight leg raise.

A. Name the muscle group acting at the hip to perform the SLR. _____

B. Name the antagonist muscle group at the hip. _____

C. As the leg is raised, select the type of contraction the hip agonist is performing.

_____ Isometric _____ Concentric
_____ Eccentric _____ None

D. As the leg is lowered, select the type of contraction the hip agonist is performing.

_____ Isometric _____ Concentric
_____ Eccentric _____ None

E. Name the muscle group acting at the knee to maintain it extended. _____

F. Name the antagonist muscle group at the knee. _____

G. As the leg is raised, select the type of contraction the knee agonist is performing.

_____ Isometric _____ Concentric
_____ Eccentric _____ None

H. As the leg is lowered, select the type of contraction the knee agonist is performing.

_____ Isometric _____ Concentric
_____ Eccentric _____ None

10. Examining the location of the biceps brachii on the anterior surface of the arm, the insertion of its tendon on the radius indicates that the biceps will flex the elbow and supinate the forearm.

A. When the elbow is in extension with the forearm supinated and the biceps performing an isometric contraction, in terms of angle of pull, what force does the biceps exert on the elbow?

_____ Approximation _____ Traction

B. When the elbow is in full flexion with the forearm supinated and the biceps performing an isometric contraction, in terms of angle of pull, what force does the biceps exert on the elbow?

_____ Approximation _____ Traction

11. Move from a sitting to a standing position.

A. The lower extremities are moving in

_____ an open kinetic chain.

_____ a closed kinetic chain.

B. Which hip and knee muscle groups are the agonists?

_____ Extensors _____ Flexors

C. The agonists are performing what type of contractions?

_____ Concentric _____ Eccentric

_____ Isometric _____ None

12. From a standing position, sit down.

A. The lower extremities are moving in

_____ an open kinetic chain.

_____ a closed kinetic chain.

B. Which muscle groups are the agonists?

_____ Extensors _____ Flexors

C. The agonists are performing what type of contractions?

_____ Concentric _____ Eccentric

_____ Isometric _____ None

■ ■ ■ Post-Lab Questions

Student's Name _____

Date Due _____

After you have completed the worksheets and lab activities, answer the following questions without using your book or notes. When finished, check your answers.

1. A. When the agonist is contracting to overcome the resistance of gravity, the body part is moving in the

   _____ same direction as the force of gravity.
   _____ opposite direction as the force of gravity.

   B. The the agonist is contracting

   _____ concentrically. _____ eccentrically.
   _____ isometrically.

2. A. When the agonist is contracting to slow down the force of gravity, the body part is moving in the

   _____ same direction as the force of gravity.
   _____ opposite direction as the force of gravity.

   B. The agonist is contracting

   _____ concentrically. _____ eccentrically.
   _____ isometrically.

3. When the agonist is contracting isotonically, the antagonist is _____·_____.

4. A. While sitting, raise your arm through full flexion range of motion. The agonists are the shoulder

   _____ flexors. _____ extensors.

   B. While sitting, lower your arm to the anatomical position from full flexion. The agonists are the shoulder

   _____ flexors. _____ extensors.

   C. While supine, raise your arm through full ROM.

   During the first half of the ROM (0–90 degrees), the agonists are the

   _____ flexors. _____ extensors.

During the second half of the ROM (90–180 degrees), the agonists are the

   _____ flexors. _____ extensors.

   D. While supine, return your arm to the anatomical position from full flexion.

   During the first half of the ROM (180–90 degrees), the agonists are the

   _____ flexors. _____ extensors.

   During the second half of the ROM (90–0 degrees), the agonists are the

   _____ flexors. _____ extensors.

5. What is the relationship between muscle fiber arrangement and the force a muscle can produce?

   _____

   _____

   _____

6. When a muscle lacks irritability, it will lack the ability to _____.

7. When the lower extremity is held at the end of the range of SLR, the hamstrings muscles have been _____. When the lower extremity is then lowered to anatomical position, the hamstrings are able to return to _____ because of the property of _____.

8. A person who has less hip flexion ROM when performing an SLR than when flexing the hip and knee simultaneously would experience _____ insufficiency of the _____.

9. In the sitting position with the upper extremity in the anatomical position, curl (flex) just your fingers as much as possible. Now flex your wrist. Which of the following may be true?

_____ A. Passive insufficiency of the finger flexors

_____ B. Passive insufficiency of the finger extensors

_____ C. Passive insufficiency of the wrist flexors

_____ D. Passive insufficiency of the wrist extensors

_____ E. Active insufficiency of the finger flexors

_____ F. Active insufficiency of the finger extensors

_____ G. Active insufficiency of the wrist flexors

_____ H. Active insufficiency of the wrist extensors

10. If the elbow joint were designed to have abduction ROM under voluntary control, what would be the location of the muscle(s) that would perform elbow abduction?

_____

_____

11. What is the relationship between types of kinetic chain and whether the origin moves toward the insertion or the insertion moves toward the origin during a muscle contraction?

_____

_____

_____

Nervous System

■ ■ ■ Pre-Lab Worksheets

Student's Name _____

Date Due _____

Complete the following questions prior to the lab class.

1. Match the following terms and descriptors.

    _____ Transmit impulses   A. Neurons
          toward cell body

    _____ Nerve cell   B. Cell body

    _____ Integrates signals   C. Myelin
          from sensory neurons

    _____ Conductor of impulses   D. Node of
          from the cell body   Ranvier

    _____ Has cell body in   E. Axon
          dorsal root ganglion

    _____ Group of myelinated   F. Dendrite
          nerve fibers within
          CNS

    _____ Distal end of axon   G. Anterior root
                                        (ventral)

    _____ Includes major tracts   H. Posterior root
          in the CNS   (dorsal)

    _____ Large cell body with   I. Interneuron
          a long axon

    _____ Contains mostly   J. Nerve fiber
          unmyelinated fibers

    _____ Has both dendrites   K. Synapse
          and an axon extending
          from it

    _____ Fatty sheath   L. Tract

    _____ Conducts nerve   M. White matter
          impulses from the
          neuron

    _____ Collection of axons   N. Gray matter
          located near the
          intervertebral foramen

    _____ Break in myelin sheath   O. Motor neuron

    _____ Gap between neurons   P. Motor endplate

    _____ Collection of dendrites   Q. Sensory neuron
          located near the
          intervertebral foramen

2. What structure connects the right and left cerebral
   hemispheres? _____

3. Complete the following table.

Lobe	Location in Brain	Main Function
Frontal		
Occipital		
Parietal		
Temporal		

4. Match the spinal cord coverings with their location.

    _____ Outer layer   A. Arachnoid
                                mater

    _____ Middle layer   B. Dura mater

    _____ Inner layer   C. Pia mater

5. Match each of the following structures with its major function.

_____ Thalamus   A. Hormone function and behavior

_____ Hypothalamus   B. Body sensations— where pain is perceived

_____ Basal ganglia   C. Automatic control of respiration

_____ Midbrain   D. Coordination of motor movement

_____ Medulla oblongata   E. Control of muscle coordination, tone, posture

_____ Cerebellum   F. Center for visual reflexes

6. A. The subarachnoid space is located between which spinal cord coverings?

_____ and _____

B. What circulates through the subarachnoid space?

_____

C. What is its function?

_____

_____

7. Match the following spinal cord elements with their descriptions.

_____ Contains neuronal cell bodies and synapses   A. Conus medullaris

_____ End of spinal cord   B. Cauda equina

_____ Collection of nerve roots   C. Filum terminale

_____ Non-neural portion of spinal cord   D. Gray matter

8. Label the drawing of vertebra using the following terms (Fig. 6-1).

Vertebral foramen   Body   Neural arch

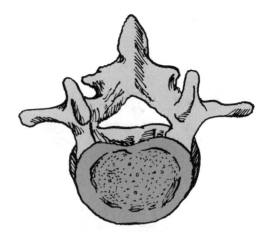

FIGURE 6-1 Vertebra, superior view.

9. Label the cross-section drawing of the spinal cord using the following terms (Fig. 6-2).

Gray matter   Posterior horn   Anterior horn
Peripheral nerve   Posterior columns   White matter
Anterior root   Posterior root

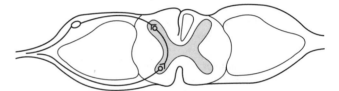

FIGURE 6-2 Spinal cord.

10. The conus medullaris is located approximately at the level of the _____ lumbar vertebra.

11. The cauda equina is made up of the nerve roots for what spinal levels? _____ .

12. The filum terminale is at which end of the spinal cord?

_____ Proximal _____ Distal

13. The corticospinal tract is the main pathway for _____ .

The tract crosses from one side of the brain to end in the opposite side of spinal cord at the level of the _____ .
The corticospinal pathways synapse in the _____ horn.

14. An upper motor neuron synapses in the anterior horn cell and is considered part of a peripheral nerve.

    _____ True _____ False

15. Match the cranial nerve name with the cranial nerve number.

    _____ Facial   A. XI

    _____ Spinal accessory   B. V

    _____ Trigeminal   C. VII

16. Indicate whether the following spinal nerves exit above or below the vertebra of the same number. If there is not a matching vertebra, indicate which vertebra it exits below.

Nerve	Above	Below	Vertebra
C1			
C7			
C8			
T1			

17. The spinal nerve divides into the posterior (dorsal) ramus and the anterior (ventral) ramus. What is the function of each ramus?

    Posterior (dorsal) ramus: _____

    Anterior (ventral) ramus: _____

18. List the major muscle groups innervated by each of the following spinal segments.

    A. C1–C3 _____

    B. C5–C6 _____

    _____

    C. C6–T1 _____

    _____

    D. T2–T12 _____

    E. L2–L4 _____

    _____

    F. L4–S3 _____

    _____

19. For each of the three major nerve plexuses, provide the spinal levels that combine to make the plexus.

    A. Cervical plexus: _____

    B. Brachial plexus: _____

    C. Lumbar plexus: _____

    Lumbar portion: _____

    Sacral portion: _____

20. On the drawing of the brachial plexus (Fig. 6-3), label the following structures:

    Cords   Nerve roots   Peripheral nerves
    Trunks   Divisions

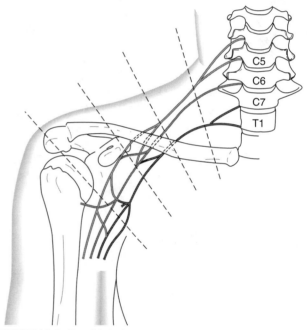

FIGURE 6-3 Brachial plexus.

21. On the drawing of the nervous system (Fig. 6-4), identify and label the following structures:

Afferent neuron   Axon terminals
Axon   Myelin sheath
Dendrites   Node of Ranvier
Efferent neuron   Cell body

22. Identify which peripheral nerve(s) arise(s) from the following nerve roots:

C5–C6: _____

C6–T1: _____

C8–T1: _____

L2–L4: _____

L4–S3: _____

L4–S2: _____

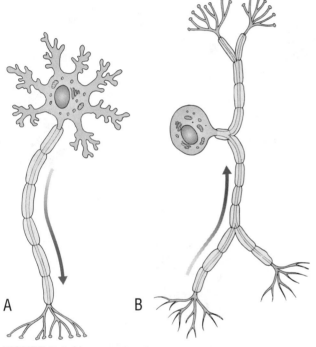

FIGURE 6-4 Neuron structure.

■ ■ ■ Lab Activities

Student's Name _____

Date Due _____

1. Using models of the brain and skull, locate the lobes of the brain. Note the relationship of the lobes within the skull.

2. Using a model of the spinal column, locate

   A. the divisions of the vertebral column—cervical, thoracic, lumbar, sacral, and coccyx.

   B. the intervertebral foramen.

3. Place stockinets on your arm and leg, then draw on the stockinet the path of the peripheral nerves and the sensory distribution of the peripheral nerves. Use the stockinets as study guides for reviewing peripheral nerves and their sensory distribution. Alternatively, you can use a washable marker or skin pencil to draw on your arm and leg. For the peripheral nerve pathways, refer to Figures 6-23 through 6-33 in the Lippert textbook, 5th edition.

   A. Upper extremity: Since the peripheral nerves emerge from the brachial plexus as the five individual nerves at approximately the head of the humerus, begin drawing at that level. Describe path and sensory distribution of each.

      1) Axillary nerve:

         a. Path: _____

         _____

         b. Sensory distribution: _____

         _____

      2) Musculocutaneous nerve:

         a. Path: _____

         _____

         b. Sensory distribution: _____

         _____

      3) Radial nerve:

         a. Path: _____

         _____

         b. Sensory distribution: _____

         _____

      4) Median nerve:

         a. Path: _____

         _____

         b. Sensory distribution: _____

         _____

      5) Ulnar nerve:

         a. Path: _____

         _____

         b. Sensory distribution: _____

         _____

   B. Lower extremity: Since the peripheral nerves emerge from the lumbosacral plexus and enter the thigh at the proximal end of the lower extremity as individual nerves, begin drawing at the inguinal ligament anteriorly, and below the buttock posteriorly.

      1) Obturator nerve:

         a. Path: _____

         _____

         b. Sensory distribution: _____

         _____

      2) Femoral nerve:

         a. Path: _____

         _____

         b. Sensory distribution: _____

         _____

      3) Sciatic nerve:

         a. Path: _____

         _____

         b. Sensory distribution: _____

         _____

      4) Tibial nerve:

         a. Path: _____

         _____

         b. Sensory distribution: _____

         _____

5) Common peroneal nerve:

a. Path: _____

_____

b. Sensory distribution: _____

_____

4. Identify the dermatome area for C5–C6.

5. Using string or yarn of different colors, construct models of the brachial and lumbar plexuses.

6. Using the skeleton, arrange string or yarn to illustrate the pathways of the peripheral nerves.

7. Palpate the ulnar nerve in the groove between the medial epicondyle and the olecranon process. When you rolled or tapped on the nerve, did you feel a "pins and needles" sensation in your little finger?

8. Describe and assume the postures resulting from the following nerve injuries. Identify the nerve involved.

Posture	Description	Nerve
Erb's palsy		
Scapular winging		
Wrist drop		
Ape hand		
Pope's blessing		
Claw hand		
Drop foot		

■ ■ ■ Post-Lab Questions

Student's Name _____

Date Due _____

After you have completed the worksheets and lab activities, answer the following questions without using your book or notes. When finished, check your answers.

1. Underline the correct response in the parentheses. Peripheral nerves have both efferent and afferent fibers. Efferent information originates in the (spinal cord/periphery) and is about (sensory/motor) function. Afferent information originates in the (spinal cord/periphery) and is about (sensory/motor) function.

2. On the following table, indicate if the structures are part of the central nervous system (CNS) or the peripheral nervous system (PNS).

Structure	CNS	PNS
Median nerve		
Brain stem		
Parietal lobe		
Anterior horn		
Corticospinal tract		
Nerve roots		
Femoral nerve		

3. Match the following movements with the peripheral nerve that innervates the muscle(s) responsible for that motion.

   _____ Forearm pronation   A. Ulnar

   _____ Shoulder abduction   B. Radial

   _____ Elbow extension   C. Musculocutaneous

   _____ Wrist ulnar deviation   D. Axillary

   _____ Elbow flexion   E. Median

4. Match the following movements with the peripheral nerve that innervates the muscle(s) responsible for that motion.

   _____ Hip adduction   A. Peroneal

   _____ Ankle dorsiflexion   B. Sciatic

   _____ Knee extension   C. Obturator

   _____ Toe flexion   D. Tibial

   _____ Hip extension   E. Femoral

5. For the major nerves that supply the upper extremity, identify the associated spinal level.

Nerve	Spinal Level
Axillary	
Musculocutaneous	
Radial	
Median	
Ulnar	

6. Match the major nerves that supply the lower extremity with the associated spinal level.

   _____ Femoral   A. L4–S3

   _____ Sciatic   B. L2–L4

7. Match each of the following impairments with the nerve injury that may cause it.

   _____ Scapular winging   A. Ulnar nerve

   _____ Wrist drop   B. Long thoracic nerve

   _____ Ape hand   C. Median nerve

   _____ Claw hand   D. Radial nerve

8. Name the two nerves that the sciatic nerve divides into.

   _____

9. When an adult sustains an injury to the nervous system at the L4–L5 level, is it a lower motor neuron injury? Why?

   _____

Circulatory System

■ ■ ■ Pre-Lab Worksheets

Student's Name _____

Date Due _____

Complete the following questions prior to the lab class.

1. The arteries of the pulmonary circuit transport
   _____ blood and the arteries of the
   systemic circuit transport _____
   blood.

2. The pulmonary circuit consists of what structures?

   _____

   The systemic system consists of what structures?

   _____

3. The heart lies within the _____
   with most of the heart on the _____
   side.

4. The ventricle with the thickest wall is the
   _____.

   Why is this ventricle wall thicker? _____

   _____

5. The valves between the atria and ventricles are called
   _____ valves. The valve
   between the right atrium and ventricle is also called
   the _____ valve. The one
   between the left atrium and ventricle has two other
   names based on number of valve flaps and shape.
   They are the _____ or
   _____ valves. The valves leaving
   the ventricles are the _____
   valves. The valve between the right ventricle and
   the pulmonary artery is also known as the
   _____ or
   _____ valve. The valve

between the left ventricle and the aorta is also
known as the _____
valve.

6. Draw a flowchart showing the path blood takes,
   beginning when it leaves the heart, continuing as it
   travels through the body, and ending at the starting
   point.

7. Heart sounds result from the forceful closing
   of _____. The "lub"
   sound comes from the closing of the
   _____ and the "dub" sound
   from the closing of the _____.

8. The cardiac cycle is what pushes the blood through
   the lungs and body. When the atria contract, blood
   moves into the _____, which in turn
   contract to push blood onward to either the
   _____ or _____.

9. What vessels form the connection between the
   arterioles and venules? _____

10. On Figure 7-1, label the following:

Coronary arteries   Brachiocephalic trunk

Ascending aorta   Descending aorta

Subclavian arteries   Common carotid
  (R & L)   arteries (R & L)

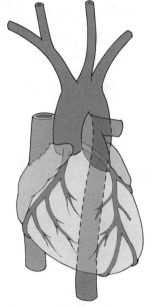

FIGURE 7-1 Arteries near the heart.

11. On Figure 7-2, label the following:

Common iliac   External iliac   Internal iliac
  arteries   arteries   arteries

Right common   Left common   Inferior vena
  iliac vein   iliac vein   cava

External iliac
  vein

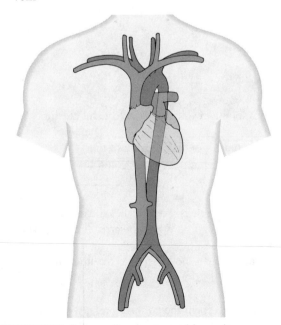

FIGURE 7-2 Descending aorta and branches.

12. The femoral artery passes through the
_____ muscle to the posterior
aspect of the knee, where the name changes to
_____.

13. Match the arteries with the areas of the CNS they
supply.

_____ Arterial system   A. External carotid
       supplying blood   arteries
       to brain

_____ Supplies the   B. Internal carotid
       occipital lobes   arteries

_____ Joins the anterior   C. Basilar artery
       and posterior
       cerebral arteries

_____ Supplies the   D. Posterior cerebral
       cerebellum, pons,   arteries
       and midbrain

_____ Joins the right   E. Circle of Willis
       and left cerebral
       arteries

_____ Supplies the   F. Posterior
       scalp, dura,   communicating
       and skull   artery

_____ Supplies the   G. Anterior
       anterior part of   communicating
       the brain   artery

14. Draw a flowchart of the arteries of the upper
extremity.

15. List the four main functions of the lymphatics:

_____

_____

_____

_____

16. The sacs that are located along the paths of lymph vessels are _____. These sacs contain _____ that help to digest the contents of the lymph. An important means of moving lymph is contraction of the smooth muscle of the _____.

17. Name the regions of the body that drain lymph into the right lymphatic duct.

_____

_____

_____

_____

18. List the three main groups of regional nodes: _____

_____

19. Lymph vessels between the clavicle and umbilicus drain into the _____ nodes.

■ ■ ■ Lab Activities

Student's Name _____

Date Due _____

1. Simulate the blood supply to the brain: Hold the index and middle fingers of each hand up in front of you. The fingers of your left hand represent the right and left vertebral arteries (posterior), and the fingers of your right hand represent the internal carotid arteries (anterior). Your forearms represent the vertebral and common carotid arteries running up the neck. Balance a ball on the top of your four fingertips. The ball represents a brain. Ask your partner to place a piece of string or yarn around your four fingertips to form the circle of Willis.

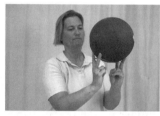

FIGURE 7-3 Simulating the circle of Willis.

2. Using a washable *red* marker, draw the major arteries of the upper and lower extremities on your partner. Using a washable *blue* maker, draw the major veins of the upper and lower extremities on your partner. Alternatively, draw the blood vessels on a stockinet placed on your partner's extremities.

   A. Draw a line from the middle of the clavicle to the middle of the cubital fossa (axillary and brachial arteries).

   B. At the inferior border of the cubital fossa, split the brachial artery into the radial and ulnar arteries that run the length of the respective bones.

3. Palpate pulses at the brachial, radial, and carotid arteries.

   A. The brachial artery pulse can be palpated on the anterior aspect of the elbow, medial to the _____ of the _____ muscle. With the use of a _____ and _____ (blood pressure cuff), this artery can be used to measure the _____. The brachial artery can be found in the anterior cubital fossa. It may be difficult to find in obese individuals or those with well-developed muscles.

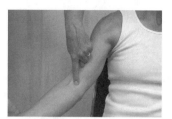

FIGURE 7-4 Palpating the brachial artery.

   B. Radial artery: With your forearm supinated, the radial artery can be found on the lateral side at the wrist. Placing your fingers parallel along the lateral side of the most lateral tendon (flexor carpi radialis), you should feel a strong pulse.

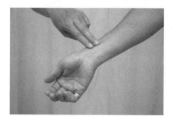

FIGURE 7-5 Palpating the radial artery.

   C. With your partner sitting and facing you, palpate the carotid artery in the space between the thyroid cartilage (Adam's apple) and the SCM muscle. Because this artery supplies much of the blood to the brain, do not palpate both sides at the same time.

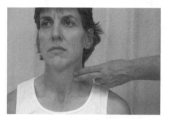

FIGURE 7-6 Palpating the carotid artery.

4. Palpate pulses in the lower extremity:

   A. The femoral artery can be found in the groin area, at the crease where your lower abdomen meets the upper thigh. Palpate midway between the ASIS to the uppermost part of the pubic symphysis (mid-inguinal point) medial to the tendon of the rectus femoris.

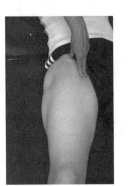

FIGURE 7-7 Palpating the femoral artery.

B. The popliteal artery can be palpated with your partner in the prone position and knee flexed approximately 90 degrees. Because the artery is deep, press your fingers into the area lateral to the medial hamstring muscles and proximal to the popliteal crease. Palpating this pulse is difficult.

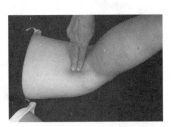

FIGURE 7-8 Palpating the popliteal artery.

C. Palpate the dorsal pedis artery by placing your fingers between the bases of the great toe and second toe and then tracing that line straight up the foot to the dorsal-most prominence of the navicular bone.

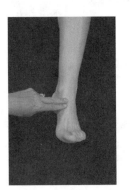

FIGURE 7-9 Palpating the dorsal pedis artery.

D. Palpate the posterior tibial artery by inverting the ankle to relax the reticulum and then placing your fingers in the groove between the posterior border of the medial malleolus and the Achilles tendon.

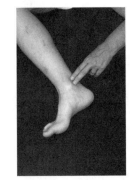

FIGURE 7-10 Palpating the posterior tibial artery.

E. The great saphenous vein is usually visible in thin males when standing. Trace it from anterior to the medial malleolus, up the medial tibia, just posterior to the medial border of the patella, and up the medial thigh to just distal to the inguinal ligament at its midpoint.

5. Blood circulation is partially responsible for maintaining body temperature. Using the back of your hand, palpate your partner from the dorsum of his or her foot to the proximal anterior thigh. Can you detect any difference in temperature of the skin in these two areas? Explain why a difference might exist.

_____

_____

6. Palpate just medial along the inferior surface of the lower jaw for lymph nodes. Often the lymph nodes in this area become enlarge when a person has a cold.

■ ■ ■ Post-Lab Questions

Student's Name _____

Date Due _____

After you have completed the worksheets and lab activities, answer the following questions without using your book or notes. When finished, check your answers.

1. Fill in the structure that performs the function listed:

Function	Structure
Prevents backflow of blood into ventricles	
Contains heart, aorta, trachea between lungs	
Only branches of ascending aorta	
Pumping chambers	
Prevents backflow of blood into atria from ventricles	
Collecting chambers	

2. What happens when the valves of the veins of the lower extremity do not close completely?

    _____

    _____

3. Organize the following list of arteries in order from distal to proximal:
    Posterior tibial   Popliteal   Dorsal pedis
    Femoral   Anterior tibial

    • _____
    • _____
    • _____
    • _____

4. The first branch of the subclavian artery is the

    _____.

5. Which arteries are typically palpated when determining heart rate? _____

    _____

6. Blood pressure is recorded as the
    _____ pressure over the
    _____ pressure.

7. The systolic pressure represents the pressure when the heart is

    _____ contracting. _____ at rest.

8. The cardiovascular system is a _____ system and the lymphatic system is a _____ system.

9. The main functions of the cardiovascular system are to

    _____.

10. The main functions of the lymphatic system are to

    _____.

11. The descending aorta branches at L4 to become the right and left _____ iliac arteries. In turn, this artery branches at approximately S1 into the _____ and _____ arteries. The _____ artery supplies the lower extremity. As this artery passes under the inguinal ligament, it becomes the _____ artery. It runs distally along the anterior and medial side of the thigh. At the lower one-third of the thigh, it passes through an opening in the adductor muscle into the _____ fossa, where it becomes the _____ artery. At the distal end of the fossa, it divides into the _____ and _____ arteries. The _____ artery emerges to descend along the anterior leg, becoming the _____ artery at the ankle. The _____ artery remains on the posterior side of the leg, and its pulse can be felt in the groove between the posterior border of the medial malleolus and the Achilles tendon.

12. Number the following structures sequentially as they are encountered by blood. Begin at the systemic venous side of the heart.

    ___ Lungs   ___ Vena cavae

    ___ Left ventricle   ___ Left atrium

    ___ Right ventricle   ___ Pulmonary artery

    ___ Aorta   ___ Pulmonic valve

    ___ Right atrium   ___ Aortic valve

    ___ Tricuspid valve   ___ Bicuspid valve

Basic Biomechanics

■ ■ ■ Pre-Lab Worksheets

Student's Name _____

Date Due _____

Complete the following questions prior to the lab class.

1. Match the following terms with their definitions.

   _____ Mechanics

   A. Application of mechanics to the study of the structure and function of the human body

   _____ Biomechanics

   B. Factors associated with moving systems

   _____ Dynamics

   C. Study of forces and the motions they produce

   _____ Statics

   D. Factors associated with nonmoving systems

2. Kinetic deals with _____ causing movement. Kinematics involves which three aspects of a moving system?

   _____

3. Osteokinematics deals with the movement of _____, and arthrokinematics deals with the movement of _____.

4. Match the following terms with their definitions.

   _____ Force

   A. Force that causes motion

   _____ Vector

   B. Describes speed

   _____ Scalar

   C. Amount of matter a body contains

   _____ Mass

   D. Tendency of force to produce rotation

   _____ Inertia

   E. Push or pull action

   _____ Kinetics

   F. Describes magnitude only

   _____ Torque

   G. Resistive force between two surfaces

   _____ Friction

   H. Magnitude and direction

   _____ Velocity

   I. Resistance to change in motion

5. Match Newton's laws of motion with the example that illustrates the law.

   _____ Law of inertia

   A. A sailboat speeds up as the wind force increases.

   _____ Law of acceleration

   B. The archer pulls back on the string and releases the arrow.

   _____ Law of action-reaction

   C. A person is pushing on a stubborn donkey trying to get it to move.

6. Draw examples of linear forces, parallel forces, and concurrent forces and include the resultant force.

7. Match the type of force with an example.

_____ Force couple   A. Two horses pulling a wagon

_____ Parallel forces   B. Tug-of-war

_____ Concurrent forces   C. Unscrewing a jar lid

_____ Linear force   D. A car stuck in the snow is freed when one person pushes forward at the middle of the back bumper and another person pushes at the passenger side door.

8. Another term for *torque* is _____. Torque is a force that produces _____ about an axis. The amount of torque produced depends on the _____ of the force and the _____ from the force's line of pull to the axis of rotation.

9. Gravity is the mutual attraction between the _____ and an _____. Gravitational force is always directed _____ to the center of the earth. Where is the center of gravity of the body considered to be located in an adult?

_____

10. In some countries, women transport objects by carrying them on top of their heads. What happens to the center of gravity when an object is carried in this manner?

_____

11. Providing an ambulatory assistive device such as a walker does what to the base of support and overall stability?

BOS: _____

Stability: _____

12. Simple machine levers have three basic components. List these components.

A. _____

B. _____

C. _____

13. Using Figure 8-1, identify the class of lever for each of the following tools and indicate the axis (A), resistance (R), and the force (F).

Implement	Class of Lever	Order of AFR
Barbecue tongs		
Pliers		
Nutcracker		

FIGURE 8-1 (A) Barbecue tongs. **(B)** Pliers. **(C)** Nutcracker.

14. List the two purposes for using a pulley.

A. _____

B. _____

15. An inclined plane exchanges _____ for _____.

16. A basic rule of simple machines is what advantage is gained in _____ is lost in _____.

■ ■ ■ Lab Activities

Student's Name _____

Date Due _____

1. You have two balls of approximately the same size: One is a soccer ball and the other is a medicine ball. Kick each ball with the same amount of force. *Use caution if you are indoors!*

   A. Which ball has more mass? _____

   B. Which ball will travel farther? _____

   C. Why? _____

   D. This is demonstrating which of Newton's laws?

   _____

   E. Which ball requires more force to move? Why?

   _____

   F. This demonstrates which of Newton's laws?

   _____

2. With your partner, perform the following activities and identify which type of force is being demonstrated.

   Linear force   Parallel force   Concurrent force
   Force couple   Resultant force

   A. Stand next to your partner, facing a table. Push the table forward. _____

   B. You and your partner stand facing each other on opposite sides of a table and push the table toward each other. _____

   C. You and your partner stand on opposite sides and ends of a table. Each of you push straight forward on the table. _____

   D. You and your partner position yourselves as illustrated in Figure 8-2, and each pulls the rope toward yourself. Try to pull with the same amount of force.

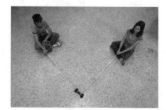

FIGURE 8-2 Starting position for Lab Activity #2D.

1) This demonstrates what type of force?

   _____

2) In which direction did the dumbbell move?

   _____

3) The direction the dumbbell moves demonstrates what type of force?

   _____

3. Analyze the type of mechanical force acting on the elbow joint in each of the following positions.

   A. With the elbow extended at your side and holding a weight in your hand, the type of mechanical force acting on the elbow is

   _____.

   B. With the elbow extended, place your hand on a table and lean on it. The type of mechanical force on the elbow is _____.

4. In a standing position while maintaining the elbow in extension and holding a weighted cuff in your hand, perform shoulder flexion. Repeat with the weighted cuff secured above the elbow. Which is easier? Why?

   _____

   _____

5. What is the effect on the body's center of gravity when the shoulder is at 90 degrees of flexion?

   _____

6. What is the effect on the body's center of gravity when the shoulder is at 180 degrees of flexion?

   _____

7. Standing with your back and legs against the wall and without flexing your knees, attempt to pick up an object on the floor about 5 inches in front of your toes.

   A. Could you pick up the object? _____

   B. Explain. _____

   _____

8. Assume the hands and knees position. Start each of the following from the hands knees position.

   • First, lift one hand off the floor.

   • Second, lift one leg off the floor.

- Third, lift one hand and the opposite leg off the floor.
- Fourth, lift the hand and leg on the same side off the floor.

A. For each of the four positions, describe the BOS and the COG.

_____

B. Which position is most stable?

_____

C. Which is most unstable?

_____

D. Explain. _____

9. Stand with one foot on each side of a doorjamb such that your forefoot is beyond the door frame and your nose touches the door frame. Rise up on your toes.

A. Could you rise up on your toes? _____

B. Explain. _____

_____

10. Assume each of the following positions and analyze the stability of each:

- On all fours (hands and knees)
- Lying down
- Kneeling
- Squatting (on balls of feet)
- Standing with feet together
- Standing with feet apart

A. Observe and describe the BOS and location of the COG in each posture.

_____

_____

_____

_____

_____

_____

B. Gently push on your partner in various directions in each of the following positions and rank them from most stable (1) to least stable (6).

_____ Down on all fours

_____ Lying supine

_____ Kneeling

_____ Squatting

_____ Standing with feet together

_____ Standing with feet apart

11. Find a partner who is the same approximate size as you. Sit on the floor with your backs against each other. At the same time, push against each other and stand up.

A. At what point did you feel most stable?

_____

B. At what point did you feel least stable?

_____

C. Why? _____

12. Sitting with your upper extremity in anatomical position, move your shoulder through full flexion range of motion so that your fingers are pointing directly overhead.

A. The starting shoulder range of motion is _____, and the ending range of motion is _____.

B. What is the "axis" of the motion? _____

C. Is the movement with or against gravity?

_____

D. Is muscle producing the force for movement or the resistance to movement? _____

E. Is gravity producing the force for movement or the resistance to movement? _____

F. Which major muscle group is the agonist?

_____

G. Is the agonist performing a concentric or an eccentric contraction? _____

H. Is the antagonist contracting? _____

13. Analyze the motion at the shoulder joint as the arm returns to anatomical position from full flexion.

A. The starting range of motion is _____, and the ending range of motion is _____.

B. What motion is being performed? _____

C. Is the movement with or against gravity?

_____

D. Is muscle producing the force for movement or the resistance to movement? _____

E. Is gravity producing the force for movement or the resistance to movement? _____

F. Which major muscle group is the agonist?

_____

G. Is the agonist performing a concentric or an eccentric contraction? _____

14. In the supine position, move your shoulder through full flexion range of motion, beginning in anatomical position. **ATTENTION:** The effect of gravity on the movement of shoulder flexion varies throughout the range.

First phase: Flex the shoulder from anatomical position until the hand is pointing to the ceiling.

A. The starting range of motion is _____, and the ending range of motion is _____.

B. Is the movement with or against gravity?

_____

C. Is muscle producing the force for movement or the resistance to movement? _____

D. Is gravity producing the force for movement or the resistance to movement? _____

E. Which major muscle group is the agonist?

_____

F. Is the agonist performing a concentric or an eccentric contraction? _____

Second phase: Flex the shoulder from midrange (the hand pointing toward the ceiling) to the end of flexion range of motion.

A. The starting range of motion is _____, and the ending range of motion is _____.

B. What is the "axis" of the motion? _____

C. Is muscle producing the force for movement or the resistance to movement? _____

D. Is gravity producing the force for movement or the resistance to movement? _____

E. Which major muscle group is the agonist?

_____

F. Is the agonist performing a concentric or an eccentric contraction? _____

15. In the supine position, extend your shoulder from full flexion.

First phase: Extend the shoulder from full flexion until the hand is pointing toward the ceiling.

A. The starting range of motion is _____, and the ending range of motion is _____.

B. Is the force producing the movement muscle or gravity? _____

C. Is the resistance to the movement muscle or gravity?

_____

D. Which muscle group is the agonist? _____

E. What type of contraction is the agonist performing? _____

Second phase: Extend the shoulder from the hand pointing toward the ceiling to the anatomical position.

A. The starting range of motion is _____, and the ending range of motion is _____.

B. Is the force producing the movement muscle or is gravity? _____

C. Is the resistance to the movement muscle or gravity? _____

D. Which muscle group is the agonist? _____

E. What type of contraction is the agonist performing? _____

16. The following activity involves sitting in a wheelchair and assessing how changes in COG and BOS affect stability and determining what happens when an inclined plane is added. For safety, have your partner stand behind the wheelchair as a spotter throughout this activity.

A. Sit in a wheelchair with your feet on the footplates:

1) Describe the BOS and location of your COG.

_____

_____

2) Add a backpack full of books or weights to the back of the wheelchair.

Did the BOS change? _____

What happened to the COG? _____

3) What happens to the COG if you add more books (weights)?

_____

B. Sit cross-legged or with your feet on the seat:

1) Did the BOS change? _____

2) What happened to the COG? _____

C. Sitting in the same position, add a backpack full of books and remove the footplates:

1) Did the BOS change? _____

2) What happened to the COG? _____

D. Replace the footplates and remove the backpack, then propel yourself up a ramp:

1) Did the BOS change? _____

2) What happened to the COG? _____

3) How did you shift your body? How did that affect COG? _____

_____

_____

E. Sitting with your feet on the footplates and a backpack full of books attached to the back of the wheelchair, propel yourself up the ramp:

1) How did you shift your body? _____

2) How did that affect COG? _____

F. Sit cross-legged with a backpack full of books attached to the back of the wheelchair and the footplates removed. Propel yourself up the ramp.

1) How did this compare to your other attempts to propel yourself up the ramp? _____

2) Explain: _____

G. In your last trip up the ramp, what tended to happen when you pushed yourself quickly as opposed to slowly? Explain. _____

17. Repeat propelling yourself up a ramp in the following ways using an amputee or a reclining-back wheelchair. Figure 8-3 shows the difference between an amputee or reclining-back wheelchair and a standard wheelchair. If an amputee wheelchair is not available, add weighted cuffs to the footplates of a standard wheelchair.

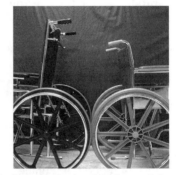

FIGURE 8-3 Standard wheelchair on right and reclining-back wheelchair on left. Note placements of axles.

• Sitting in the wheelchair with feet on footplates
• Sitting in the wheelchair without footplates and feet on seat
• Sitting in chair with feet in seat and with backpack on back of chair

A. How has the BOS changed with an amputee or reclining back wheelchair?

_____

_____

_____

B. Did propelling yourself up the ramp any of the three times feel unstable? Explain.

_____

_____

_____

■ ■ ■ Post-Lab Questions

Student's Name _____

Date Due _____

After you have completed the worksheets and lab activities, answer the following questions without using your book or notes. When finished, check your answers.

1. Describe a stable object in terms of BOS and COG.

   _____

2. A person riding a bus stands facing the front of the bus. How should the person place his or her feet to maintain balance when

   A. the bus stops?

   _____

   B. the bus turns a corner?

   _____

3. What happens to the COG when a person holds a 20-pound weight in the left hand?

   _____

   To compensate for the 20-pound weight, in which direction does a person shift the COG?

   _____

4. What happens to the COG when a person holds that 20-pound weight in both hands directly over the head?

   _____

5. Match the following terms with their definitions.

   _____ Inertia   A. Tendency of a force to produce rotation about an axis

   _____ Torque   B. Vector that describes speed

   _____ Friction   C. Resistance to any change of its motion in either speed or direction

   _____ Velocity   D. Force that tends to prevent motion of one surface across another

6. When people injure some part of their lower extremity, they are often provided with crutches to keep the body weight off the injured leg. How do the crutches affect stability?

   _____

7. For each class of lever, identify the relationship of the axis, resistance arm, and force arm, and name a tool that uses that lever class (tool example may vary).

   A. First class: _____

   B. Second class: _____

   C. Third class: _____

8. While standing, perform hip flexion, first with the knee flexed and then with the knee extended. Which knee position requires the most hip flexor strength, flexed or extended? _____

   Why? _____

9. When the force arm is longer than the resistance arm, is it easier or harder to move?

   _____

10. Describe how the angle of pull of the elbow flexors can create an angular force, a stabilizing force, or a dislocating force.

    _____

    _____

    _____

11. Moment arm or torque arm is the _____ distance from the line of action of the _____ to the _____ of rotation. The moment arm of a muscle is greatest when the line of pull of a muscle is at _____.

12. In Figure 8-4, the person in the kayak is using the paddle as a lever. Identify the axis, force, and resistance.

_____

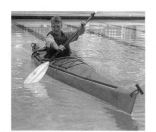

FIGURE 8-4 Kayaker paddling.

13. Label each of the following examples with the appropriate explanation of Newton's law of motion.

   A. A person with a complete spinal cord injury (SCI) at C5 is in a manual wheelchair race with a person with a complete SCI at T10. The wheelchairs and the weight of the racers are equal. Because of the level of injury, the upper extremity strength of the person with a SCI at T10 will be greater compared to the person with the SCI at C5. Which of Newton's laws explains why the person with a T10 SCI is likely to win?

   _____

   B. A person with weakness of the left shoulder muscles is sitting with the shoulder and elbow in the anatomical position. A weighted cuff is placed around the person's left wrist with instructions to lift the arm and weight ten times. In addition to weakness making this a challenging exercise, which of Newton's laws explains why initiating the movement is difficult? _____

   C. Tossing a weighted ball against a trampoline is an example of a plyometric exercise. When the ball is caught upon its return, rather than stopping the ball immediately, one grasps the ball and moves the arm in the same direction as the ball is moving. Which of Newton's laws explains the rebound of the ball off the trampoline? _____

Clinical Kinesiology and Anatomy of the Upper Extremities

Shoulder Girdle

Student's Name _____

Date Due _____

Complete the following questions prior to the lab class.

1. In the table, indicate which bones make up each of the structures.

Structures	Scapula	Clavicle	Sternum	Rib Cage	Humerus
Shoulder complex					
Scapulothoracic articulation					
Shoulder girdle					
Shoulder joint					

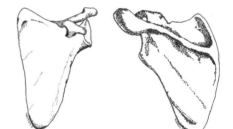

2. Define the following terms:

   Scapulohumeral rhythm: _____

   _____

   _____

   Reversal of muscle action: _____

   _____

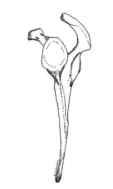

   _____

3. Label Figures 9-1 to 9-3 with the following terms:

   SCAPULA: Superior angle   Inferior angle
            Vertebral border   Axillary border
            Spine   Coracoid process
            Acromion process   Glenoid fossa

FIGURE 9-1 Landmarks of the scapula.

CLAVICLE: Sternal end   Acromial end   Body   SKULL: Occipital protuberance

STERNUM: Manubrium   Body   VERTEBRA: Spinous process   Transverse
         Xiphoid process Sternal notch   process

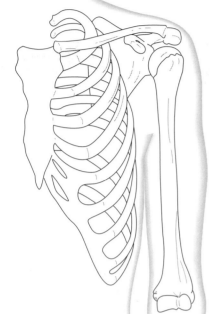

FIGURE 9-2 Landmarks of the clavicle and sternum.

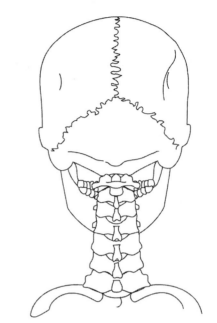

FIGURE 9-3 Landmarks of the skull and cervical spine.

4. On Figure 9-4A and B:

   A. Label the joints and bones.

   BONES: Sternum   Clavicle   Ribs
            Coracoid   Acromion   Scapula
            process

JOINTS: Sternoclavicular   Acromioclavicular

B. Label the following structures:

Sternoclavicular ligament   Costoclavicular ligament
Coracoacromial ligament   Acromioclavicular ligament
Coracoclavicular ligament   Articular disk

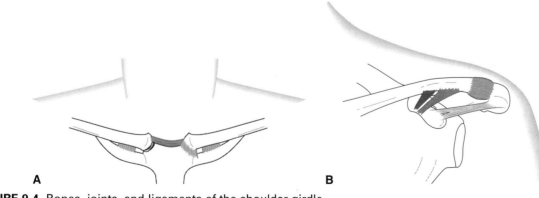

A   **B**

FIGURE 9-4 Bones, joints, and ligaments of the shoulder girdle.

5. On Figures 9-5 through 9-8:

A. Label the origin and insertion of the muscle(s) listed. Color the origin in red and the insertion in blue.

B. Join the origin and insertion to show the line of pull.

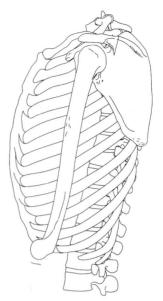

FIGURE 9-7 Serratus anterior.

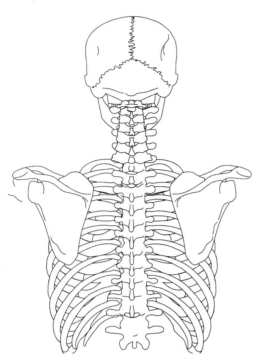

FIGURE 9-5 Upper trapezius, middle trapezius, and lower trapezius.

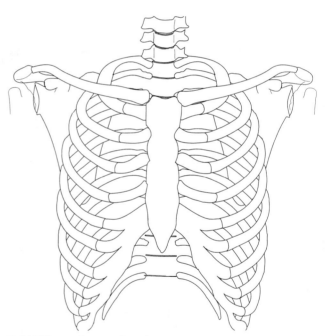

FIGURE 9-8 Pectoralis minor.

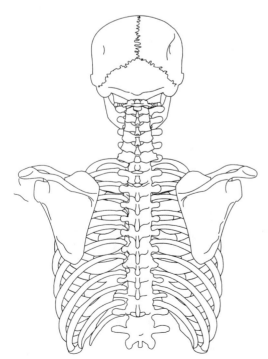

FIGURE 9-6 Levator scapula and rhomboids.

6. Draw in the muscles that make up the force couples acting on the scapula to produce upward rotation in Figure 9-9 and downward rotation in Figure 9-10. Label the muscles involved.

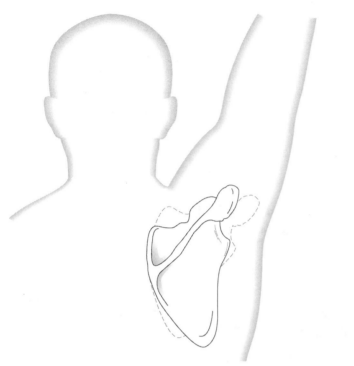

FIGURE 9-9 Upward rotation of the scapula.

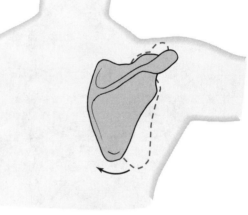

FIGURE 9-10 Downward rotation of the scapula.

7. Identify the shoulder girdle motions illustrated in Figure 9-11.

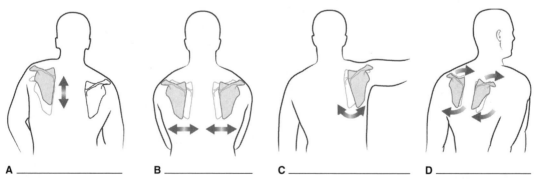

A _____   B _____   C _____   D _____

FIGURE 9-11 Shoulder girdle motions.

8. Match each ligament or structure to the appropriate function. There may be more than one correct answer, and answers may be used more than once.

_____ Connects sternum to clavicle
    A. Sternoclavicular ligament

_____ Connects first rib to clavicle
    B. Costoclavicular ligament

_____ Connects clavicles
    C. Articular disk

_____ Connects scapula to clavicle
    D. Interclavicular ligament

_____ Reinforces the capsule
    E. Acromioclavicular ligament

_____ Limits clavicular elevation
    F. Coracoacromial ligament

_____ Acts as a shock absorber

_____ Limits clavicular depression

_____ Serves as roof over humeral head

_____ Provides protective arch

9. For each motion listed, check the muscles that are the major contributors to the motion.

Motions	Upper Trapezius	Middle Trapezius	Lower Trapezius	Rhomboids	Serratus Anterior	Pectoralis Minor	Levator Scapula
Elevation							
Depression							
Protraction							
Retraction							
Upward rotation							
Downward rotation							

10. At the sternoclavicular joint, identify which surface is concave and which is convex.

Joint	Concave	Convex
Sternoclavicular		

11. With the possible exception of scapular tilt, in which plane do the motions of scapula occur?

_____

12. In an erect posture, scapular elevation is moving with/against gravity and is produced by a _____ contraction of the _____ and _____ muscles.

■ ■ ■ Lab Activities

Student's Name _____

Date Due _____

1. Palpation of bones and landmarks, ligaments, and other structures:
   • Locate on bones, skeleton, and your lab partner.
   • The reference position is the anatomical position.
   • Not all structures can be palpated on your partner.

Sternum:	Located midline of the anterior chest wall **FIGURE 9-12** Palpation of the sternum.
Manubrium:	The superior portion of the sternum **FIGURE 9-13** Palpation of the manubrium.
Body:	The middle and largest portion of the sternum **FIGURE 9-14** Palpation of the body of the sternum.
Xiphoid process:	The inferior portion of the sternum. The most inferior part of the xiphoid process is called the *tip of the xiphoid.* **FIGURE 9-15** Palpation of the xiphoid process.
Sternal notch:	The indentation at the top of the manubrium formed by the right and left clavicles and the manubrium. Palpate the sternum starting at the sternal notch, and moving inferiorly, palpate in turn the manubrium, body, and xiphoid process. **FIGURE 9-16** Palpation of the sternal notch.
Clavicle:	Located on the anterior surface of the trunk, superior and lateral to the sternum. Palpate starting at the sternal notch and moving horizontally, laterally, and posteriorly along the clavicle to the acromioclavicular joint. Note that the medial two-thirds is convex and the lateral one-third is concave. **FIGURE 9-17** Palpation of the clavicle.

Continued

Scapula:	Located superiorly on the posterior surface of the trunk between T2 and T7
Vertebral border:	The medial edge of the scapula, which is approximately parallel to the vertebral column. Palpate from superior to inferior. Medially rotating the shoulder joint by placing the hand on the lower back often causes the vertebral border to move away from the thorax.

FIGURE 9-18 Palpation of the vertebral border.

Inferior angle:	The inferior point of the scapula where the vertebral and axillary borders meet

FIGURE 9-19 Palpation of the inferior angle.

Axillary border:	The lateral edge of the scapula. The axillary border, also called the *lateral border,* becomes difficult to palpate because the latissimus dorsi, teres major, and teres minor muscles cover the border. Palpate by moving superiorly along the lateral border of the scapula from the inferior angle.

FIGURE 9-20 Palpation of the axillary border.

Acromion process:	The flat, broad expansion of the spine of the scapula that articulates with the clavicle and forms the top of the shoulder. The tip of the acromion is often used as a landmark for measurements of the upper extremity. The tip of the acromion is the anterior lateral aspect of the acromion.

FIGURE 9-21 Palpation of the acromion process.

Spine of the scapula:	A ridge or spine about one-third of the way down from the superior border of the scapula. The acromion process is the lateral end. The medial end on the vertebral border of the scapula is a flat, smooth triangle called the *root* or *base* of the spine of the scapula. Palpate by moving posteriorly, medially, and inferiorly from the acromion process to the vertebral border. 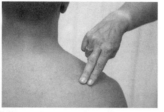 **FIGURE 9-22** Palpation of the spine of the scapula.
Superior angle:	The angle formed as the vertebral border of the scapula joins the superior border. Palpate by moving superiorly from the root of the spine of the scapula. The superior angle is difficult to palpate because it is deep to the levator scapula and trapezius muscles.
Coracoid process:	The projection on the anterior surface of the scapula. Palpate from the anterior surface of the trunk inferior to the acromioclavicular joint. Deep to the pectoralis major muscle, the coracoid process can be palpated by pressing deeply into the tissues. This may be uncomfortable for the individual being palpated. 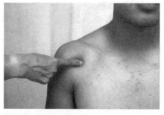 **FIGURE 9-23** Palpation of the coracoid process.

2. Palpation of muscles:

A. Locate the following muscles on the skeleton, anatomical models, and on at least one partner.

- The information needed to palpate each muscle is provided in the following tables.
- The position described for locating the muscle on your partner is usually the manual muscle test position for a fair or better grade of muscle strength.
- Not all origins, insertions, and muscle bellies can be palpated on your partner.

B. On the skeleton, locate the origin and insertion of each muscle.

- Place the ends of a rubber band at the origin and insertion of the muscle, making the band taut. Note the location of the muscle in relation to the joints it crosses.
- When possible, move the skeleton to perform the muscle's motion and observe how the band becomes less taut, similar to the change in length as it performs a concentric contraction.

Sitting Position

UPPER TRAPEZIUS:	Located superficially on the posterior thorax
Position of person:	Sit facing away from the examiner with hands relaxed in the lap **FIGURE 9-24** Palpation of the upper trapezius.
Origin:	Occipital protuberance and nuchal ligament of upper cervical spinous processes
Insertion:	Outer third of clavicle and acromion process
Line of pull:	Diagonal (more vertical than horizontal)

Continued

Sitting Position—Cont'd

Muscle action:	Prime mover in scapular elevation and upward rotation and only assistive in scapular retraction
Palpate:	On the superior and posterior aspect of the thorax above the scapula
Instructions to person:	Shrug or raise your shoulder toward your ear.
LEVATOR SCAPULA:	Located on the posterior thorax deep to the upper trapezius. Its location and the fact that it has similar action to the upper trapezius makes it difficult to palpate.
Position of person:	Sit facing away from the examiner with the hands relaxed in the lap
Origin:	Transverse processes of C1–C4 vertebrae
Insertion:	Vertebral border of scapula between the superior angle and the root of the spine
Line of pull:	Diagonal line of pull that is mostly vertical
Muscle action:	Prime mover for scapular elevation and downward rotation, and assistive in scapular retraction
Palpate:	On the posterior surface of the thorax at the superior angle of the scapula
Instructions to person:	Shrug your shoulder toward your ear.
PECTORALIS MINOR:	Located on the anterior chest wall deep to the pectoralis major

FIGURE 9-25 Palpation of the pectoralis minor.

Position of person:	Sit facing the examiner with the hand of the side being palpated resting on the lower back.
Origin:	Anterior medial outer surfaces of ribs 3–5
Insertion:	Coracoid process of the scapula
Line of pull:	Diagonal (downward pull is mostly vertical)
Muscle action:	Prime mover for scapular depression, downward rotation, and tilt
Palpate:	Below the coracoid process
Instructions to person:	Lift your hand off your lower back.
SERRATUS ANTERIOR:	Located on the anterior lateral chest wall deep to the latissimus dorsi laterally and deep to the scapula posteriorly

FIGURE 9-26 Palpation of the serratus anterior.

Position of person:	Sit with the shoulder flexed to 90°.
Origin:	Lateral aspects of first eight ribs
Insertion:	Anterior surface of the vertebral border of the scapula
Line of pull:	Horizontal
Muscle action:	Prime mover for scapular protraction and upward rotation
Palpate:	On the anterior lateral aspect of the chest wall
Instructions to person:	Reach forward with your shoulder flexed by protracting your scapula.

Prone Position

LOWER TRAPEZIUS:	Located superficially on the posterior thorax

FIGURE 9-27 Palpation of the lower trapezius.

Position of person:	Lie prone with the shoulder abducted to approximately 145° (in line with the fibers of the muscle).
Origin:	Spinous processes of middle and lower thoracic vertebrae
Insertion:	Base of the spine of the scapula
Line of pull:	Diagonal (mostly downward)
Muscle action:	Prime mover for scapular depression and upward rotation; also assists in retraction
Palpate:	The muscle belly inferior and medial to the insertion
Instructions to person:	Lift your arm off the table toward the ceiling.

MIDDLE TRAPEZIUS:	Located superficially on the posterior thorax

FIGURE 9-28 Palpation of the middle trapezius.

Position of person:	Lie prone with shoulder abducted to 90° and the elbow flexed to 90°. The forearm should be hanging over the edge of the table.
Origin:	Spinous processes of C7–T3
Insertion:	Medial aspect of the acromion process and spine of the scapula

Line of pull:	Horizontal
Muscle action:	Prime mover for scapular retraction and assistive for upward rotation
Palpate:	Lateral to the origin
Instructions to person:	Lift your upper arm off the table toward the ceiling.

RHOMBOIDS:	Located on the posterior thorax deep to the trapezius
Position of person:	Lie prone with hand resting on the lower back
Origin:	Spinous processes of C7–T5 vertebrae
Insertion:	Vertebral border of scapula between the spine and the inferior angle of the spine
Line of pull:	Diagonal
Muscle action:	Prime mover in scapular retraction, elevation, and downward rotation
Palpate:	Medial to the vertebral border of the scapula
Instructions to person:	Lift your hand off your lower back toward the ceiling.

3. Perform the motions of the shoulder girdle with your partner.

   A. Perform a motion and have your partner name the motion you performed.

   _____

   B. Your partner calls a motion and you perform that motion.

   _____

4. Observe and palpate as your partner flexes her or his shoulder, starting in the anatomical position.

   A. List the scapular motion(s) you observed.

   _____

   B. Place one hand along the vertebral border. Palpate the movement of the scapula as your partner repeats shoulder flexion. Describe what you felt.

   _____

C. Stabilize the scapula to prevent its movement by placing one hand on the acromion process and the other along the axillary boarder as your partner attempts shoulder flexion. Describe what you observed.

_____

_____

5. Observe and palpate as your partner performs shoulder abduction starting in the anatomical position.

A. Describe the movements of the scapula and humerus in relation to one another.

_____

_____

B. What is the name given to this combination of movements?

_____

6. Work in groups of at least three. Have one person stand in functional position. Have the second partner place a heavy weight in the first person's right hand, while the third person palpates the right shoulder girdle musculature.

A. What happened to the shoulder girdle (e.g., elevation or depression) on the side holding the weight?

_____

_____

B. Name any shoulder girdle musculature that contracted in response to the weight.

_____

_____

C. What force is the weight exerting on the shoulder girdle?

____ Traction ____ Approximation

D. What type of kinetic chain activity is this?

____ Open ____ Closed

E. Perform shoulder elevation on the side holding the weight.

1) The shoulder elevator muscles are ___ overcoming gravity ___ slowing down gravity.

2) What type of contractions are the muscles performing?

____ Concentric _____ Eccentric

7. A. When your partner assumes the hands-and-knees position, what position do her or his scapulae assume? Circle the correct answer.

Neutral   Protracted   Retracted   Winged

B. What type of kinetic chain activity is this?

____ Open ____ Closed

C. What muscle keeps the scapula close to the ribs?

_____

8. **Functional activity analysis:**

In each chapter on the upper extremity, you will be analyzing the activity of placing a plate in a cabinet then removing the plate and placing it on the counter. Perform those tasks and then describe the position of the person's scapula in Figures 9-29 and 9-30.

_____

_____

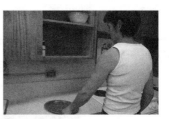

FIGURE 9-29 Starting position of placing plate in cabinet; end position for removing plate from cabinet.

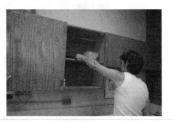

FIGURE 9-30 Starting position of placing plate on counter; end position for placing plate in cabinet.

■ ■ ■ Post-Lab Questions

Student's Name _____

Date Due _____

After you have completed the worksheets and lab activities, answer the following questions without using your book or notes. When finished, check your answers.

1. List the shoulder girdle muscle(s) that attach to the ribs.

   _____

2. List the shoulder girdle muscle(s) that attach to the vertebral border of the scapula.

   _____

3. List the shoulder girdle muscle(s) that attach to the skull.

   _____

4. List the shoulder girdle muscle(s) that attach to the vertebral column.

   _____

5. List the shoulder girdle muscle(s) that attach to the clavicle.

   _____

6. List the joint(s) that make up the shoulder girdle.

   _____

7. Why is the scapulothoracic joint not a true joint?

   _____

8. What is the result of limited sternoclavicular motion on shoulder girdle motion?

   _____

9. Using the following descriptive terminology, fill in the blanks in the following sentences. Use each term once.

   Medial   Anterior   Superior   Deep
   Lateral   Posterior   Inferior   Superficial

   A. The spine is on the _____ surface of the scapula.

   B. The vertebral border is on the _____ side of the scapula.

   C. The glenoid fossa is on the _____ aspect of the scapula.

   D. The xiphoid process is _____ to the body of the sternum.

   E. The rhomboid muscles are located _____ to the trapezius.

   F. The coracoid process is on the _____ surface of the scapula.

   G. The upper trapezius muscle is _____ to the levator scapula.

   H. The clavicle is _____ to the first rib.

10. Identify the following muscles:

    A. Attaches to the coracoid process: _____

    B. Attaches to the vertebral border of the scapula:

       1) On the posterior surface: _____

       2) On the anterior surface: _____

    C. Attaches to the superior angle of the scapula: _____

    D. Attaches to the spine of the scapula:

       _____

    E. Attaches at the base of the spine:

       _____

    F. Attaches on the transverse processes of the vertebra: _____

    G. Attaches on the spinous process of the vertebra: _____

11. Identify the following muscles according to their locations on the body:

    A. Which muscle is located between the rib cage and the scapula? _____

    B. Which muscle lies deep to the pectoralis major? _____

    C. Which muscle is the most superficial on the posterior upper back? _____

12. Name the muscle innervated by a cranial nerve: _____

    Name the cranial nerve: _____

Shoulder Joint

Student's Name _____

Date Due _____

Complete the following questions prior to the lab class.

1. On Figure 10-1A and B, label the following landmarks:

SCAPULA:	Glenoid fossa	Labrum
	Subscapular fossa	Infraspinous fossa
	Supraspinous fossa	Axillary border
	Acromion process	Vertebral border
HUMERUS:	Head	Surgical neck
	Anatomical neck	Shaft
	Greater tubercle	Lesser tubercle
	Deltoid tuberosity	Bicipital groove

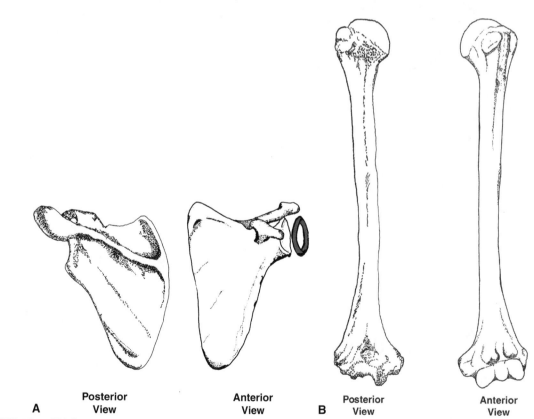

	A		**B**	
	Posterior View	**Anterior View**	**Posterior View**	**Anterior View**

FIGURE 10-1 **(A)** Scapula, anterior and posterior views. **(B)** Humerus, anterior and posterior views.

2. On Figure 10-2:

 A. Label the shoulder joint and bones.

 B. Label the following structures:

Glenohumeral ligaments   Coracohumeral ligament

Greater tubercle   Capsule

Tendon of long head
 of biceps

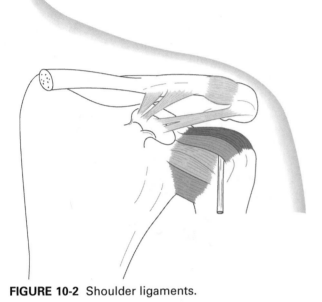

FIGURE 10-2 Shoulder ligaments.

3. On Figures 10-3 through 10-7:

 A. Label the origin and insertion of the muscles listed.

 B. Join the origin and insertion to show the line of pull.

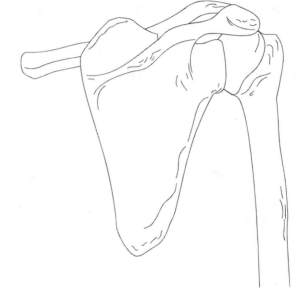

FIGURE 10-3 Supraspinatus, infraspinatus, teres minor, and triceps—long head proximal attachment.

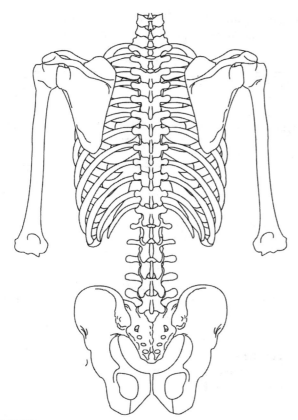

FIGURE 10-4 Latissimus dorsi and teres major.

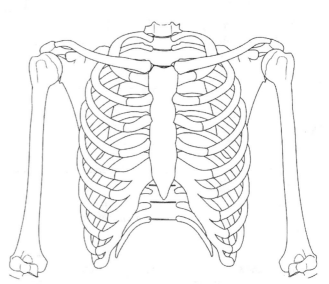

FIGURE 10-6 Pectoralis major and coracobrachialis.

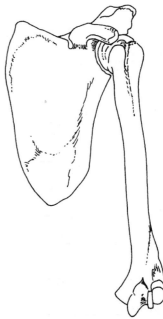

FIGURE 10-7 Subscapularis and proximal attachments of biceps.

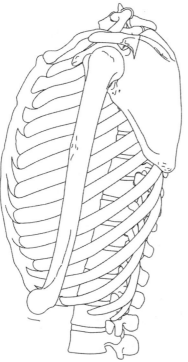

FIGURE 10-5 Anterior deltoid, middle deltoid, and posterior deltoid.

4. Describe the role of scapulohumeral rhythm and the "inchworm effect" in maintaining the effectiveness of the shoulder muscles.

_____

_____

_____

_____

5. Distinguish between the shoulder joint and the shoulder girdle by *listing the bones* of each.

Shoulder Joint	Shoulder Girdle

6. Distinguish between the shoulder joint and the shoulder girdle by *listing the motions* available at each.

Shoulder Joint	Shoulder Girdle

7. For the shoulder joint, identify the following:

A. Type of joint: _____

B. Shape of the joint: _____

8. For the motions available at the shoulder joint, indicate in which plane and about which axis motion occurs.

Motions	Plane	Axis
Flexion/extension/ hyperextension		
Abduction/adduction		
Medial/lateral rotation		

9. Identify which surface of the shoulder joint is concave and which is convex.

Joint	Concave	Convex
Shoulder joint		

10. For the shoulder joint, provide the close-packed position and the loose-packed position (refer to Chapter 4, Table 4-4).

Joint	Close-Packed	Loose-Packed
Shoulder		

11. Match each ligament and structure to the appropriate function or characteristic. Use each answer once.

_____ Provides attachment for the latissimus dorsi muscle   A. Coracohumeral ligament

_____ Deepens the joint   B. Glenoid labrum

_____ Keeps the humeral head rotating in contact with the glenoid fossa   C. Subdeltoid bursa

_____ Surrounds the joint   D. Subacromial bursa

_____ Strengthens the upper part of the joint capsule   E. Rotator cuff

_____ Decreases friction between the deltoid muscle and the joint capsule   F. Thoracolumbar fascia

_____ Decreases friction between the acromion process, the coracoacromial ligament, and the joint capsule   G. Joint capsule

12. For each motion listed, check the muscle(s) that are major contributors to the motion.

Motion	Anterior Deltoid	Middle Deltoid	Posterior Deltoid	Supraspinatus	Coracobrachialis	Subscapularis
Flexion						
Extension						
Hyperextension						
Medial rotation						
Lateral rotation						
Abduction						
Adduction						
Horizontal abduction						
Horizontal adduction						

Motion	Pectoralis Major Clavicular	Pectoralis Major Sternal	Latissimus Dorsi	Teres Major	Teres Minor	Infraspinatus
Flexion						
Extension						
Hyperextension						
Medial rotation						
Lateral rotation						
Abduction						
Adduction						
Horizontal abduction						
Horizontal adduction						

13. Describe the function of the rotator cuff muscles during shoulder flexion or abduction.

_____

_____

_____

14. A. Which major nerve unit is located in the axilla? _____

B. That nerve unit is where in relation to the head of the humerus?

_____ Anterior _____ Posterior

_____ Superior _____ Inferior

C. What major blood vessel is close to this nerve unit? _____

■ ■ ■ Lab Activities

Student's Name —————————————————

Date Due ————————————————————

1. Palpation of bones and landmarks, ligaments and other structures:
   • Locate on bones, skeleton, and your lab partner.
   • The reference position is the anatomical position.
   • Not all structures can be palpated on your partner.

Scapula*

Glenoid fossa	A shallow socket on the superior end, lateral side; it articulates with the humerus. Cannot be palpated.
Glenoid labrum	Fibrocartilaginous ring attached to the rim of the glenoid fossa, which deepens the articular cavity. Cannot be palpated.
Subscapular fossa	Includes most of the area on the anterior surface; provides attachment for the subscapularis muscle. Cannot be palpated.
Infraspinous fossa	Area on the posterior surface, below the spine; provides attachment for the infraspinatus muscle. Cannot be palpated.
Supraspinous fossa	Area on the posterior surface, above the spine; provides attachment for the supraspinatus muscle. Cannot be palpated.
Axillary border	Lateral aspect, provides attachment for teres major and teres minor muscles. See Figure 9-20.
Acromion process	Broad, flat area on the superior lateral aspect of the scapula; it provides attachment for the middle deltoid muscle. See Figure 9-21.

*Some of the landmarks on the scapula were described in the lab on the shoulder girdle (Chapter 9).

Humerus

Head	Smooth, semiround portion of the proximal end medial aspect of the humerus. The head of the humerus fits in the glenoid fossa to complete the shoulder joint. The head is palpable when the shoulder joint is laterally rotated. 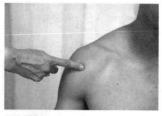 **FIGURE 10-8** Palpating head of the humerus.
Surgical neck	Slightly constricted area just distal to the tubercles where the head meets the body of the humerus. Cannot be palpated.
Anatomical neck	Circumferential groove separating the head from the tubercles. Cannot be palpated.
Shaft	Extends from the surgical neck proximally to the epicondyles distally. Also known as the body of the humerus.
Greater tubercle	Large projection on the proximal end of the humerus lateral to head and lesser tubercle. It provides attachment for the supraspinatus, infraspinatus, and teres minor muscles. Palpate the greater tubercle on your partner by finding the tip of the acromion process and sliding distally onto the greater tubercle of the humerus. A second method is palpating the proximal anterior surface of the humerus while medially rotating the humerus. This movement causes the greater tubercle to move under your fingers. 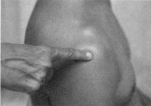 **FIGURE 10-9** Palpating the greater tubercle.

Continued

Humerus—Cont'd

Lesser tubercle	Smaller projection on the proximal anterior surface of the humerus medial to the greater tubercle; it provides attachment for the subscapularis muscle. Palpate the lesser tubercle on your partner by placing your fingers on the proximal anterior surface of the humerus medial to the greater tubercle while laterally rotating the humerus with your other hand. This movement causes the lesser tubercle to move under your fingers.
Deltoid tuberosity	Located laterally at the midpoint of the shaft of the humerus. The deltoid muscle inserts on the deltoid tuberosity. It is not a well-defined structure, and it is not easily palpated. **FIGURE 10-10** Palpating the deltoid tuberosity.
Bicipital groove	Located between the tubercles on the proximal anterior surface of the humerus. Also called the intertubercular groove. Palpate the bicipital groove on your partner by placing your fingers on the proximal anterior surface of the humerus. Medial and lateral rotation causes the greater and lesser tubercles to move under your fingers. The space between the tubercles is the bicipital groove. The biceps tendon lies in the bicipital

groove. Palpation of the groove may produce discomfort when too much pressure is applied.

FIGURE 10-11 Palpating the bicipital groove.

Bicipital ridges	Also called the lateral and medial lips of the bicipital groove, or the crests of the greater and lesser tubercles. The lateral lip (crest of the greater tubercle) provides attachment for the pectoralis major, and the medial lip (crest of the lesser tubercle) provides attachment for the latissimus dorsi and teres major.

2. Palpation of muscles:

A. Locate the following muscles on the skeleton, anatomical models, and on at least one partner.

   • The information needed to palpate each muscle is provided in the following tables.

   • The position described for locating the muscle on your partner is usually the manual muscle test position for a fair or better grade of muscle strength.

   • Not all origins, insertions, and muscle bellies can be palpated on your partner.

B. On the skeleton, locate the origin and insertion of each muscle.

   • Place the ends of a rubber band at the origin and insertion of the muscle, making the band taut. Note the location of the muscle in relation to the joints it crosses.

   • When possible, move the skeleton to perform the muscle's motion and observe how the band becomes less taut, similar to the change in length as it performs a concentric contraction.

Sitting Position

ANTERIOR DELTOID:	Located superficially and anterior to the shoulder joint

FIGURE 10-12 Anterior deltoid.

Position of person:	Sitting facing the examiner with the arm relaxed at the side
Origin:	Lateral third of the clavicle
Insertion:	Deltoid tuberosity
Line of pull:	Mostly vertical
Muscle action:	Prime mover for horizontal adduction when the shoulder is abducted to 90°
	In anatomical position, prime mover for flexion, abduction, and medial rotation
Palpate:	Approximately 2 inches distal to the lateral clavicle
Instructions to person:	Abduct (or flex) your shoulder.
MIDDLE DELTOID:	Located superficially and superior to the shoulder joint

FIGURE 10-13 Middle deltoid.

Position of person:	Sitting facing the examiner with the arm relaxed at the side
Origin:	Acromion process
Insertion:	Deltoid tuberosity
Line of pull:	Vertical
Muscle action:	Prime mover for abduction

Palpate:	Approximately 2 inches distal to the acromion process on the lateral aspect of the humerus
Instructions to person:	Raise your arm out to the side. (You can add resistance in the direction of adduction.)
POSTERIOR DELTOID:	Located superficially and posterior to the shoulder joint

FIGURE 10-14 Palpating the posterior deltoid.

Position of person:	Sitting facing away from examiner, arm relaxed at side
Origin:	Spine of the scapula
Insertion:	Deltoid tuberosity
Line of pull:	When shoulder is abducted to 90°, line of pull is primarily horizontal. When shoulder is in anatomical position, line of pull is mostly vertical.
Muscle action:	Shoulder abduction, extension, hyperextension, lateral rotation, and horizontal abduction
Palpate:	On the posterior surface of the shoulder joint
Instructions to person:	Raise your arm to the side and to the back. (You can add resistance in the direction of flexion.)
SUPRASPINATUS:	Located deep to the upper trapezius

FIGURE 10-15 Palpating the supraspinatus.

Continued

Sitting Position—Cont'd

Position of person:	Sitting facing away from the examiner with the arm relaxed at the side
Origin:	Supraspinous fossa of the scapula
Insertion:	Greater tubercle of the humerus
Line of pull:	Horizontal
Muscle action:	Prime mover for shoulder abduction. Contributes to stabilizing head of humerus in glenoid fossa.
Palpate:	This muscle is difficult to palpate because it is deep to the upper trapezius. The muscle belly is superior to the spine of the scapula in the supraspinatus fossa.
Instructions to person:	Start to raise your arm out to the side. (You can add resistance in the direction of adduction.)
CORACOBRACHIALIS:	Located deep to the anterior deltoid and the pectoralis major, and anterior to the shoulder joint

FIGURE 10-16 Palpating the coracobrachialis.

Position of person:	Sitting facing the examiner with the arm relaxed at the side
Origin:	Coracoid process of the scapula
Insertion:	Medial surface of the humerus near the midpoint of the shaft
Line of pull:	Vertical
Muscle action:	Stabilizes the shoulder and assists with flexion and adduction

Palpate:	This muscle is difficult to palpate because it is deep to other shoulder muscles. Palpate on the proximal medial aspect of the humerus. A method to isolate the muscle is to place the person's hand on the hip, and while the person isometrically adducts the shoulder joint, palpate on the anterior medial surface of the proximal humerus. Another method is to palpate origin on the coracoid process.
Instructions to person:	Starting with the hand on hip, press your hand into hip.
LATISSIMUS DORSI:	Located superficially on the posterior thorax

FIGURE 10-17 Palpating the latissimus dorsi.

Position of person:	Prone with the arm medially rotated at the side
Origin:	Spinous process of T7–L5 via dorsolumbar fascia, posterior surface of the sacrum, iliac crest, and lower three ribs
Insertion:	Medial floor of the bicipital groove of the humerus
Line of pull:	Mostly vertical
Muscle action:	Prime mover for shoulder extension, hyperextension, medial rotation, and adduction. With the upper extremity fixed, it lifts the pelvis.
Palpate:	On the side of the thorax near the axillae, while giving resistance to shoulder adduction/extension

Sitting Position—Cont'd

Instructions to person:	Extend your shoulder as I resist you. Another method is to place your hand on your lower back and reach across toward your opposite hip.

Prone Position

TERES MAJOR:	Located superficially posteriorly between the scapula and humerus

FIGURE 10-18 Palpating the teres major.

Position of person:	Lie prone with the arm medially rotated at the side
Origin:	Axillary border of the scapula near the inferior angle
Insertion:	Crest of the humerus just inferior to the lesser tubercle and next to the insertion of the latissimus dorsi muscle
Line of pull:	Diagonal
Muscle action:	Prime mover for shoulder extension, medial rotation, and adduction
Palpate:	On the lateral border of the scapula below the axillae
Alternative method:	In the prone position, abduct the shoulder joint to 90° with the elbow flexed over the edge of the table so that the forearm is off the table and pronated. Medially rotate the shoulder joint by raising the palm of the hand toward the ceiling. Palpate the muscle belly lateral and superior to the inferior angle of the scapula.

Instructions to person:	Place your hand on your lower back and reach across your back toward your opposite hip.
INFRASPINATUS:	Located mostly superficially on the scapula with some parts deep to the middle and lower trapezius

FIGURE 10-19 Palpating the infraspinatus.

Position of person:	Lie prone with the shoulder at 90° of abduction and the elbow flexed over the edge of the table
Origin:	Infraspinous fossa of scapula
Insertion:	Greater tubercle of the humerus
Line of pull:	Mostly horizontal
Muscle action:	Prime mover for lateral rotation and horizontal abduction and assistive for extension
Palpate:	Over the infraspinous fossa below the spine of the scapula
Instructions to person:	Raise the back of your hand toward the ceiling.
TERES MINOR:	Located on the posterior scapula, mostly superficial with some parts deep to the trapezius and deltoid
Position of person:	Lie prone with the shoulder at 90° of abduction and the elbow flexed over the edge of the table
Origin:	Axillary border of the scapula
Insertion:	Greater tubercle of the humerus
Line of pull:	Diagonal
Muscle action:	Prime mover for lateral rotation and horizontal abduction

Continued

Prone Position—Cont'd

Palpate:	Palpate origin along the axillary border of the scapula. Palpate muscle belly on posterior shoulder joint.
Instructions to person:	Raise your hand so the back of your hand is toward the ceiling.

Supine Position

SUBSCAPULARIS:	Located deep in the axillae

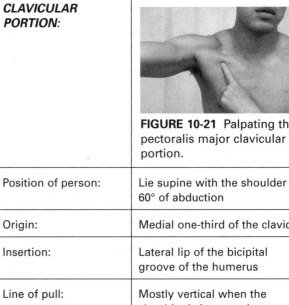

FIGURE 10-20 Palpating the subscapularis.

Position of person:	Lie supine with the arm at the side and the elbow flexed to 90º
Origin:	Anterior surface of scapula in the subscapular fossa
Insertion:	Lesser tubercle of the humerus
Line of pull:	Horizontal
Muscle action:	Prime mover for medial rotation
Palpate:	At the insertion, or in the axillae anterior to the latissimus dorsi
Instructions to person:	Pull your hand to your abdomen while I resist the motion.

PECTORALIS MAJOR— CLAVICULAR PORTION:	Located superficially on the anterior thorax

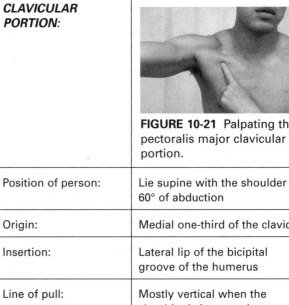

FIGURE 10-21 Palpating the pectoralis major clavicular portion.

Position of person:	Lie supine with the shoulder in 60° of abduction
Origin:	Medial one-third of the clavicle
Insertion:	Lateral lip of the bicipital groove of the humerus
Line of pull:	Mostly vertical when the shoulder is in extension
Muscle action:	Prime mover of flexion to 60°. With the sternal portion, it contributes to adduction, medial rotation, and horizontal adduction.
Palpate:	Just below the clavicle
Instructions to person:	Raise your arm across your body toward the opposite shoulder.
PECTORALIS MAJOR— STERNAL PORTION:	Located superficially on the anterior thorax

FIGURE 10-22 Palpating the pectoralis major sternal portion.

Supine Position—Cont'd

Position of person:	Lie supine with the shoulder in 120° of abduction
Origin:	Sternum and costal cartilage of the first six ribs
Insertion:	Lateral lip of the bicipital groove of the humerus
Line of pull:	Mostly vertical when shoulder is in full flexion
Muscle action:	Prime mover of shoulder extension against resistance-gravity or other force from full flexion (180°) to about 120°. With the clavicular portion, it contributes to adduction, medial rotation, and horizontal adduction.
Palpate:	At the origin or at the lower anterior border of the axillae
Instructions to person:	Move your arm across your body toward the opposite hip.

3. Perform the motions of the shoulder joint with your partner.

   A. Perform a motion and your partner names the motion you performed.

   B. Your partner states a motion and you perform that motion.

4. Using worksheet Question 8 for reference, for each of the motions available at the shoulder joint:

   A. Place your open left hand in the correct orientation to represent the plane of a motion.

   B. Place your right index finger to indicate the axis of that plane of motion.

5. Knowing the amount of motion at a joint is important for planning interventions and determining change. The normal amount of motion for each plane of motion at a joint is known. Being able to estimate the amount of joint motion present is useful. The anatomical position is considered the 0° position for most joints and is the starting position for measuring the amount of motion available in each plane. To begin estimating the amount of joint motion, identify the landmark degrees of 0°, 45°, 90°, 135°, and 180°. A right angle is 90°. Halfway between 0° and 90° is 45°; 135° degrees is halfway between 90° and 180°.

   A. Move the arms of the goniometer to each of the following angles: 0°, 45°, 90°, 135°, and 180°.

   B. Without using a goniometer, place your partner's arm in 0°, 45°, 90°, 135°, and 180° of shoulder flexion.

   C. For each of the motions available at the shoulder joint, estimate the degrees of motion available by checking the box that *most closely* describes that motion. (Do not use a goniometer.)

Motions	0°–45°	46°–90°	91°–135°	136°–180°
Flexion				
Hyperextension				
Abduction				
Horizontal abduction*				
Horizontal adduction*				
Medial rotation**				
Lateral rotation**				

*Starting position: shoulder abducted to 90°.

**Starting position: elbow flexed to 90°.

6. Being able to determine the end feel of a joint is part of an examination. With your partner in sitting or supine position, move the shoulder joint through the available range of motion. At the end of the range of motion in each plane of motion, observe the end feel. Repeat with several people. Refer to Chapter 4 for descriptions of end feel. What end feel(s) for motions of the shoulder joint did you observe?

_____ Bony_____ Soft tissue stretch
_____ Soft tissue approximation

7. First, using an anatomical model and then on your partner, place your right hand over the left shoulder joint such that your thumb is on the lesser tubercle and your index, middle, and ring fingers are close together across the greater tubercle. Identify the insertion of the muscle that is under each:

Thumb: _____

Index finger: _____

Middle finger: _____

Ring finger: _____

These muscles are collectively known as the _____ muscles.

8. Use a disarticulated skeleton or anatomical model of the shoulder joint and apply the rules of joint arthrokinematics and the concave-convex rule to perform the following activities.

A. The head of the humerus is _____ concave _____ convex.

B. The glenoid fossa is _____ concave _____ convex.

C. Observe the movement of the head of the humerus on the glenoid fossa. Circle the motions that you observed.

Spin   Roll   Glide   None

D. Observe the movement of the distal end of the humerus in relation to the movement of the proximal end of the humerus as you move the head of the humerus on the glenoid fossa. In relation to the proximal end of the humerus, the distal end moved in the _____ same direction _____ opposite direction.

E. List the muscles that assist the head of the humerus to move in the glenoid fossa without impingement against the acromion.

_____

9. Stand in the anatomical position and hold a backpack in one hand with the elbow extended.

A. The force acting on the shoulder joint is _____ approximation _____ traction.

B. Name the muscles acting at the shoulder joint to counteract the force produced by the backpack: _____

C. Name the muscles acting at the shoulder girdle to counteract the force produced by the backpack: _____

10. A person with zero strength of the elbow extensors can extend the elbow under specific conditions. In a long sitting position with arms laterally rotated and hands placed on the supporting surface slightly posterior and lateral to the trunk, the pectoralis major muscle can extend the elbow.

A. This position and movement of the upper extremities is a(an) _____ open chain activity _____ closed chain activity.

B. Explain how the pectoralis major muscle extends the elbow in the position described.

_____

_____

C. Can this be accomplished if the hand is not anchored?

_____ Yes _____ No

11. **Functional activity analysis:**

In each chapter on the upper extremity, you will be analyzing the activity of placing a plate in a cabinet then removing the plate and placing it on the counter. Perform those tasks and then analyze how the subject in Figures 10-23 and 10-24 performed those tasks.

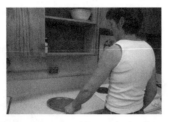

FIGURE 10-23 Starting position of placing plate in cabinet.

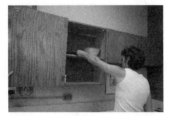

FIGURE 10-24 Starting position of placing plate on counter.

A. Describe the positions of the shoulder joint when the subject is:

1) starting to remove plate from the cabinet shelf. _____

_____

2) placing the plate on the counter. _____

_____

B. Which shoulder joint muscle groups are acting as:

1) the plate is being lowered from the cabinet shelf to the counter? _____

_____

2) the plate is being raised from the counter to the cabinet shelf? _____

_____

C. Describe the type of muscle contraction being used and why as:

1) the plate is being lowered from the cabinet shelf to the counter. _____

_____

2) the plate is being raised from the counter to the cabinet shelf. _____

_____

■ ■ ■ Post-Lab Questions

Student's Name _____

Date Due _____

After you have completed the Worksheets and Lab Activities, answer the following questions without using your book or notes. When finished, check your answers.

1. When performing shoulder flexion in an open kinetic chain, the moving part of the joint is _____ concave _____ convex.

2. You are to treat a house painter who fell off a ladder. In addition to sustaining an anterior dislocation of the shoulder, he has axillary nerve damage. Which muscle(s) may be weakened because of the nerve injury?

   _____

3. You are palpating the coracoid process and thinking about the muscle(s) attached to it. List the shoulder joint muscle(s) attaching to the coracoid process.

   _____

4. You are palpating the bicipital groove and thinking about the muscles attached on either side.

   A. List the muscle(s) attached to the lateral side of the bicipital groove:

   _____

   B. List the muscle(s) attached to the medial side of the bicipital groove:

   _____

5. A. The teres major and minor muscles attach along the _____ border of the scapula.

   B. The teres _____ muscle is located superior to the teres _____ muscle along the scapular border identified in A.

   C. The teres _____ muscle remains on the posterior surface of the shoulder while the teres _____ muscle crosses to the anterior surface.

   D. The _____ muscle, running vertically, passes between the teres major and minor in the axilla.

6. The rotator cuff muscles insert deep to the _____ muscle.

7. The _____ muscle is responsible for shoulder hyperextension.

8. The _____ muscle is inferior to the supraspinatus muscle, superior to the teres minor, and, in part, deep to the trapezius and deltoid muscles.

9. While palpating the borders of the axilla, you are thinking that the anterior border is formed by the _____ muscle and the posterior border is formed by the _____ muscle.

10. While palpating the acromion process, you are thinking that the _____ muscle passes inferior to the acromion process.

11. The nerve that innervates the deltoid muscle is often injured when the shoulder dislocates.

    A. Identify the nerve: _____

    B. Describe the sensory area innervated by this nerve: _____

12. Analyze the activity of shoulder abduction performed while standing, starting in the anatomical position.

    A. The starting range of motion is _____, and the ending range of motion is _____.

    B. What is the "axis" of the motion? _____

    C. Is the movement with or against gravity? _____

    D. Is the muscle producing the force for movement or the resistance to the movement? _____

    E. Is gravity producing the force for the movement or the resistance to the movement? _____

    F. Which major muscle group is the agonist? _____

    G. Is the agonist acting to overcome gravity or to slow down gravity? _____

    H. Is the agonist performing a concentric or an eccentric contraction? _____

    I. Is this an open or closed kinetic chain activity? _____

Elbow Joint

Student's Name _____

Date Due _____

Complete the following questions prior to the lab class.

1. Define the following term:
   Carrying angle: _____

2. On Figures 11-1 through 11-4, label the following bones and landmarks:

SCAPULA: Infraglenoid tubercle   Supraglenoid tubercle

HUMERUS: Trochlea   Capitulum
           Medial   Lateral
             epicondyle   epicondyle
           Lateral   Olecranon
             supracondylar   fossa
             ridge

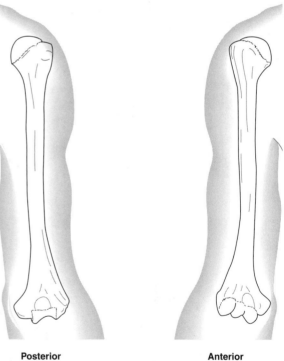

Posterior   **Anterior**

FIGURE 11-2 Landmarks of the humerus.

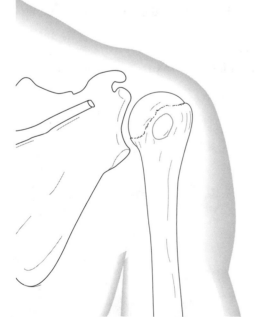

FIGURE 11-1 Landmarks of the scapula, posterior view (acromion has been removed).

ULNA: Olecranon   Trochlear   Coronoid   RADIUS: Head   Radial tuberosity   Styloid
        process   notch   process   process

       Radial   Ulnar   Styloid
        notch   tuberosity   process

       Head

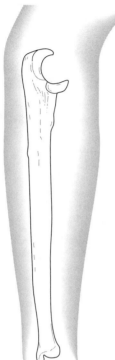

FIGURE 11-3 Landmarks of the ulna.

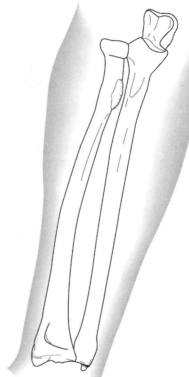

FIGURE 11-4 Landmarks of the radius.

3. On Figure 11-5, label the joints and bones of the elbow complex:

Humerus   Ulna   Radius

Elbow joint   Proximal radioulnar joint

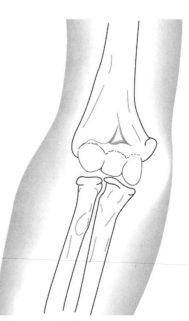

FIGURE 11-5 Bones and joints of the elbow complex.

4. On Figure 11-6, label the following structures:

Medial collateral   Lateral collateral
  ligament   ligament
Annular   Interosseous
  ligament   membrane
Capsule   Radius   Ulna

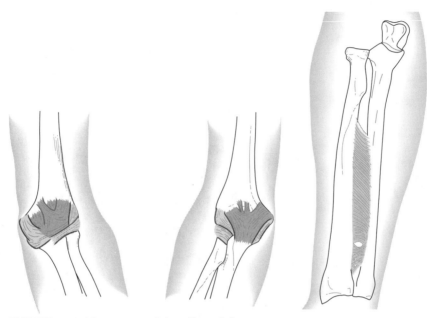

FIGURE 11-6 Ligaments of the elbow joint.

5. The motions available at the proximal and distal radioulnar joints are the _____ same or _____ different.

6. For the following joints, identify the shape of the joint, the degrees of freedom, the motions, the plane, and the axis.

Joint	Shape of Joint	Degrees of Freedom	Motions	Plane	Axis
Elbow					
Radioulnar					

7. At each of the following joints, identify which surface is concave and which is convex.

Joint	Concave	Convex
Elbow		
Radioulnar		

8. On Figures 11-7 through 11-10:

A. Label the origin and insertion of the muscles listed. Color the origin in red and the insertion in blue.

B. Join the origin and insertion to show the line of pull.

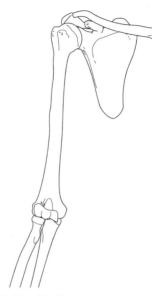

FIGURE 11-9 Brachialis.

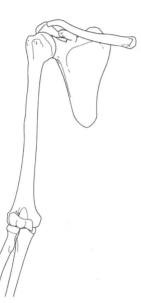

FIGURE 11-7 Biceps brachii.

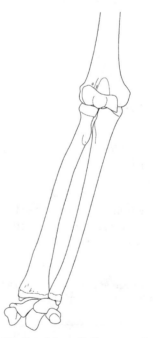

FIGURE 11-10 Brachioradialis, pronator teres, and pronator quadratus.

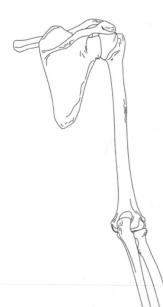

FIGURE 11-8 Triceps brachii and supinator.

9. For each of the joints below, provide the close-packed position and the loose-packed position (refer to Chapter 4, Table 4-4).

Joint	Closed-Packed	Loose-Packed
Elbow		
Radioulnar		

10. For each of the following joints, describe the end feel (refer to Chapter 4).

Joint	Bony	Soft Tissue Stretch	Soft Tissue Approximation
Elbow			
Radioulnar			

11. Match each ligament and structure to the appropriate function or characteristic. Some answers may be used more than once. Some functions or characteristics may have more than one answer.

_____ Attaches to humeral epicondyle and lateral side of ulna

A. Medial collateral ligament

_____ Is triangular in shape

B. Lateral collateral ligament

_____ Is ring-shaped

C. Annular ligament

_____ Keeps lateral side of joint from separating when stressed

D. Interosseous membrane

_____ Keeps medial side of joint from separating when stressed

E. Joint capsule

_____ Keeps radius and ulna in contact

_____ Strengthens joint capsule

_____ Attaches to humerus, radius, and ulna

12. Perform a push-up from the prone position. Analyze the elbow action of the *down* motion.

A. Is the movement with or against gravity?

_____

B. Is the muscle producing the force for the movement or the resistance to the movement?

_____

C. Is gravity producing the force for the movement or the resistance to the movement?

_____

D. Which major muscle group is the agonist?

_____

E. Is the agonist acting to overcome gravity or to slow down gravity? _____

F. Is the agonist performing a concentric or an eccentric contraction? _____

G. Is this an open or closed kinetic chain activity?

_____

■ ■ ■ Lab Activities

Student's Name _____

Date Due _____

1. Palpation of bones, landmarks, ligaments, and other structures:
   - Locate on bones or skeleton and your partner.
   - The reference position is the anatomical position.
   - Not all structures can be palpated on your partner.

Scapula

Infraglenoid tubercle	Raised portion on the inferior lip of the glenoid fossa; provides attachment of the long head of the triceps muscle. It is located deep in the joint and cannot be palpated.
Supraglenoid tubercle	Raised portion on the superior lip of the glenoid fossa; provides attachment for the long head of the biceps brachii muscle. It is located deep to the acromion process and cannot be palpated.
Coracoid process	Projection on the anterior surface, provides attachment for the short head of the biceps brachii. Palpate on the proximal anterolateral chest wall under the clavicle. Deep to the pectoralis major muscle, the coracoid process can be palpated by pressing deeply into the tissue. This may be uncomfortable for the person being palpated. See Figure 9-23.

Humerus

Trochlea	Located at the medial side of the distal end; articulates with the ulna. This structure is within the joint and thus cannot be palpated.
Capitulum	Located on the lateral side of the distal end next to the trochlea; articulates with the head of the radius. This structure is within the joint and thus cannot be palpated.
Medial epicondyle	Palpate on the medial side of the distal end of the humerus above the trochlea; larger and more prominent than the lateral epicondyle; it provides attachment for the pronator teres muscles. FIGURE 11-11 Palpating the medial epicondyle.
Lateral epicondyle	Can be observed and palpated on the lateral side of the distal end of the humerus above the capitulum; provides attachment for the anconeus and supinator muscles. FIGURE 11-12 Palpating the lateral epicondyle.
Lateral supracondylar ridge	Palpate above the lateral epicondyle; provides attachment for the brachioradialis muscle. FIGURE 11-13 Palpating the lateral supracondylar ridge.

Continued

Humerus—Cont'd

Olecranon fossa	Located on the posterior distal surface of the humerus between the medial and lateral epicondyles; articulates with the olecranon process of the ulna. Because it is deep to the triceps and olecranon process, it can be difficult to palpate. Flexing the elbow to about 90° moves the olecranon process out of the fossa without causing the triceps to become taut. This may allow the fossa to be palpated just above the olecranon process posteriorly. 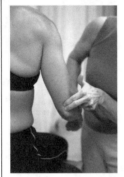 **FIGURE 11-14** Palpating the olecranon fossa.

Ulna

Olecranon process	Large prominent point of the elbow posteriorly. Palpate on the posterior proximal end of the ulna; forms the prominent point of the elbow and provides attachment for the triceps muscle. 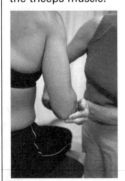 **FIGURE 11-15** Palpating the olecranon process.

Trochlear notch	Located on the anterior surface of the proximal end; articulates with the trochlea of the humerus. This structure is located within the joint and thus cannot be palpated.
Coronoid process	Located on the anterior surface of the proximal end distal to the trochlear notch; provides attachment for the brachialis muscle. Located deep to muscles. Cannot be palpated.
Radial notch	Located on the proximal end of the lateral side just distal to the trochlear notch; articulation point for the head of the radius. Located deep to muscles. Cannot be palpated.
Ulnar tuberosity	Below the coronoid process; provides attachment for the brachialis muscle. Located deep to muscles. Cannot be palpated.
Styloid process	Palpate on the distal end on the posterior medial surface. **FIGURE 11-16** Palpating the ulnar styloid process.
Head	The distal end; the ulnar notch of the radius pivots around it during pronation and supination. Cannot be palpated.

Radius

Head	Palpate on the proximal lateral aspect of the radius; articulates with the capitulum of the humerus. Hold your partner's forearm flexed at the elbow. Place the fingers of your other hand on the lateral aspect of the forearm just distal to the elbow joint. You should feel the head move under your fingers as you pronate and supinate the forearm. 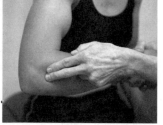 **FIGURE 11-17** Palpating the head of the radius.
Radial tuberosity	Located distal to the head on the medial side near the proximal end; provides attachment for the biceps brachii muscle. Located deep to muscles and cannot be palpated.
Styloid process	Palpate on the posterior lateral side of the distal end of the radius; provides attachment for the brachioradialis muscle. Not as prominent as the ulnar styloid process.

FIGURE 11-18 Palpating the radial styloid process.

Ligaments/Structures

Medial collateral ligament	Palpate on the medial side of the elbow; attaches on the medial epicondyle of the humerus and the coronoid process and olecranon process of the ulna.
Lateral collateral ligament	Palpate on the lateral side of the elbow; attaches on the lateral epicondyle of the humerus, the annular ligament, and the lateral side of the ulna.
Annular ligament	Encircles the head of the radius; attaches anteriorly and posteriorly to the radial notch of the ulna. Located deep to muscles and cannot be palpated.
Interosseous membrane	Between the radius and ulna. Located deep to muscles and thus cannot be palpated.

2. Palpation of muscles:

   A. Locate the following muscles on the skeleton, anatomical models, and on at least one partner.

   - The information needed to palpate each muscle is provided in the following tables.
   - The position described for locating the muscle on your partner is usually the manual muscle test position for a fair or better grade of muscle strength.
   - Not all origins, insertions, and muscle bellies can be palpated on your partner.

   B. On the skeleton, locate the origin and insertion of each muscle.

   - Place the ends of a rubber band at the origin and insertion of the muscle, making the band taut. Note the location of the muscle in relation to the joint(s) it crosses.
   - When possible, move the skeleton to perform the muscle's motion and observe how the band becomes less taut, similar to the change in length as it performs a concentric contraction.

Sitting or Standing Position

BRACHIALIS:	Located on the anterior surface of the arm, deep to the biceps brachii

FIGURE 11-19 Palpating the brachialis.

Position of person:	Facing the examiner with the arm at the side and the forearm supinated
Origin:	Anterior surface of the distal half of the humerus
Insertion:	Coronoid process and ulna tuberosity of the ulna
Line of pull:	Vertical on the anterior surface
Muscle action:	Flexes the elbow
Palpate:	Press your fingers deep on either side of the biceps tendon at the distal end of the humerus
Instructions to person:	Keeping your palm up, bend your elbow.
BRACHIORADIALIS:	Located superficially on the lateral aspect of the forearm

FIGURE 11-20 Palpating the brachioradialis.

Position of person:	Facing the examiner with the arm at the side and the forearm in the midposition, halfway between supination and pronation
Origin:	Lateral supracondylar ridge of the humerus
Insertion:	Distal lateral aspect of the radius just proximal to the radial styloid process
Line of pull:	Vertical on the anterior surface
Muscle action:	Flexes the elbow
Palpate:	Just distal to the elbow joint on the lateral side over the muscle belly
Instructions to person:	Keeping the thumb up, bend your elbow, and resist any movement with your other hand.
BICEPS BRACHII:	Located superficially on the anterior aspect of the humerus

FIGURE 11-21 Palpating the distal tendon of the biceps brachii.

Position of person:	Facing the examiner with the arm at the side and the forearm supinated
Origin:	Long head: Supraglenoid tubercle of the scapula Short head: Coracoid process of the scapula
Insertion:	Radial tuberosity of the radius

Sitting or Standing Position—Cont'd

Line of pull:	Vertical at the elbow joint and diagonal at the proximal radioulnar joint
Muscle action:	Flexes the elbow and supinates the forearm
Palpate:	The origin of the long head cannot be palpated at its origin but can be palpated in the bicipital groove. The origin of the short head can be palpated just below its attachment on the coracoid process.
Instructions to person:	Keeping your palm up, bend your elbow.
SUPINATOR:	Located deep on the lateral aspect of the elbow

FIGURE 11-22 Palpating the supinator.

Position of person:	Facing the examiner with the arm at the side and the forearm in the midposition
Origin:	Lateral epicondyle of the humerus and posterior lateral aspect of the adjacent ulna
Insertion:	Anterior surface of the proximal radius
Line of pull:	Diagonal and posterior to the joint
Muscle action:	Supinates the forearm
Palpate:	On the lateral aspect of the elbow
Instructions to person:	Turn your palm up.

PRONATOR TERES:	Located superficially on the medial aspect of the elbow

FIGURE 11-23 Palpating the pronator teres muscle.

Position of person:	Sit with the arm at the side, the elbow flexed to 90°, and the forearm in the midposition
Origin:	Medial epicondyle of the humerus and coronoid process of the ulna
Insertion:	Lateral aspect of the radius at the midpoint of the shaft
Line of pull:	Diagonal and anterior to the joint
Muscle action:	Pronates the forearm—turns the palm down
Palpate:	On the anterior surface of the proximal third of the forearm between the origin and insertion. Resisting the pronation may make the muscle easier to find.
Instructions to person:	Turn your palm down as I resist you.
PRONATOR QUADRATUS:	Located deep on the anterior distal surface of the forearm
Position of person:	Sit with the arm at side, the elbow flexed to 90°, and the forearm in the midposition
Origin:	Anterior surface of the distal quarter of the ulna
Insertion:	Anterior surface of the distal quarter of the radius
Line of pull:	Horizontal on the anterior surface

Continued

Sitting or Standing Position—Cont'd

Muscle action:	Pronates the forearm—turns the palm down
Palpate:	The pronator quadratus may be difficult to palpate because it is deep to many tendons of the wrist and hand muscles.
Instructions to person:	Turn your palm down.

Prone Position

TRICEPS BRACHII:	Located superficially on the posterior surface of the humerus

FIGURE 11-24 Palpating the triceps brachii.

Position of person:	Lie prone with the shoulder abducted to 90° and the elbow flexed over the edge of the table
Origin:	Long head: Infraglenoid tubercle of the scapula Lateral head: Inferior to the greater tubercle on the posterior side of the humerus Medial head: Posterior surface of the humerus
Insertion:	Olecranon process of the ulna
Line of pull:	Vertical on the posterior surface
Muscle action:	Extends the elbow
Palpation:	Palpate the posterior surface of the humerus
Instructions to person:	Raise your hand toward the ceiling.

ANCONEUS:	Located superficially on the posterior aspect of the elbow
Position of person:	Lie prone with the shoulder abducted to 90° and the elbow flexed over the edge of the table
Origin:	Lateral epicondyle of the humerus
Insertion:	Lateral and inferior to the triceps on the olecranon process of the ulna
Line of pull:	Diagonal and posterior to the joint
Muscle action:	Assists in extending the elbow
Palpation:	This small muscle is not present in all individuals and is difficult to separate from the triceps
Instructions to person:	Raise your hand toward the ceiling.

3. Support your partner's forearm with one hand while you *gently* palpate the structure in the groove between the medial epicondyle and olecranon process. What is this structure?

_____

4. Use a disarticulated skeleton or anatomical model of the elbow joint and apply the rules of joint arthrokinematics and the concave-convex rule to perform the following activities.

A. Underline the correct answer.
The ulna is concave /convex.
The radius is concave/convex.
The medial surface of the distal humerus is concave/convex.
The lateral surface of the distal humerus is concave/convex.

B. Move the distal bones, the radius and ulna, on the proximal bone, the humerus, in all planes of motion.

C. Observe the movement of the distal bones, the radius and ulna, on the proximal bone, the humerus. Circle the motion(s) that you observed.

Roll   Spin   Glide

D. Observe the movement of the distal ends of the radius and ulna in relation to the movement of the proximal end of the radius and ulna as you move the bones on the humerus. In relation to the proximal ends of the radius and ulna, as the elbow is flexed, the distal ends move in the _____ same direction _____ opposite direction.

E. Move the proximal bone, the humerus of the elbow joint, on the distal bones, the radius and ulna, as would occur in a closed kinetic chain activity.

F. Observe the movement of the distal end of the humerus on the radius and ulna during a closed kinetic chain activity. Circle the motions you observe.

Roll   Spin   Glide

G. In relation to the proximal end of the humerus during this movement, the distal end moves in the _____ same direction _____ opposite direction as the proximal end of the humerus during movement at the elbow joint in a closed kinetic chain activity?

5. Consider the function of the triceps muscle:

A. Position your partner prone with the shoulder abducted to 90° and the elbow flexed over the edge of the table. Palpate the triceps as your partner extends the elbow, first with the forearm supinated and then with the forearm pronated. Did the position of the forearm affect which part of the triceps contracted? Explain.

_____

_____

B. In the same starting position as in A and after your partner has extended her or his elbow, try to flex the elbow. Did the position of the forearm affect the strength of the elbow extensors? Explain.

_____

6. Consider the elbow flexor muscles: In the sitting position, place your partner's elbow at 90° of elbow flexion with the shoulder in anatomical position. Vary the position of the forearm from supinated, pronated, and midposition. In each position, ask your partner to hold the elbow flexed as you try to extend the elbow. Did the position of the forearm affect the strength of the elbow flexors? Explain your answer.

_____

_____

_____

_____

_____

_____

7. Stabilize the distal humerus with one hand and grasp the distal forearm with the other hand. Gently attempt to move the forearm into adduction. Which side of the joint is being approximated and which side is being distracted? Name the structure that limits the motion.

_____

_____

8. **Functional activity analysis:**

In each chapter on the upper extremity, you will be analyzing the activity of placing a plate in a cabinet then removing the plate and placing it on the counter. Perform those tasks and then analyze how the subject in Figures 11-25 and 11-26 performed those tasks.

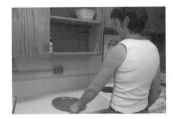

FIGURE 11-25 Starting position of placing plate in cabinet.

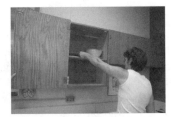

FIGURE 11-26 Starting position of placing plate on counter.

A. Describe the positions of the elbow when the subject is:

1) starting to remove the plate from the cabinet shelf. _____

2) placing the plate on the counter. _____

B. Which elbow muscle groups are acting as

1) the plate is being lowered from the cabinet shelf to the counter? _____

2) the plate is being raised from the counter to the cabinet shelf? _____

C. Describe the type of muscle contraction being used and why as

1) the plate is being lowered from the cabinet shelf to the counter. _____

2) the plate is being raised from the counter to the cabinet shelf. _____

D. Describe the positions of the forearm when the subject is

1) starting to remove plate from the cabinet shelf. _____

2) placing the plate on the counter. _____

E. Which forearm muscle groups are acting as

1) the plate is being lowered from the cabinet shelf to the counter? _____

2) the plate is being raised from the counter to the cabinet shelf? _____

F. Describe the type of muscle contraction being used and why as

1) the plate is being lowered from the cabinet shelf to the counter. _____

2) the plate is being raised from the counter to the cabinet shelf. _____

■ ■ ■ Post-Lab Questions

Student's Name _____

Date Due _____

After you have completed the worksheets and lab activities, answer the following questions without using your book or notes. When finished, check your answers.

1. Name the ring-shaped ligament within which the head of the radius rotates:

   _____

2. You are palpating the arm of a person who sustained an anterior dislocation of the elbow.

   A. Name the muscle that lies deep to the biceps brachii near the distal end of the humerus.

   _____

   B. Name the muscle that lies deep to the biceps brachii at the shoulder.

   _____

3. Name the nerve that lies in the groove between the medial epicondyle and the olecranon process.

   _____

4. Match the nerve with the muscle it innervates. Nerves may be used more than once.

   _____ Biceps brachii   A. Musculocutaneous

   _____ Triceps brachii   B. Radial

   _____ Pronator teres   C. Median

   _____ Pronator quadratus

   _____ Supinator

   _____ Brachialis

   _____ Brachioradialis

5. Which elbow flexors attach to the:

   radius? _____

   ulna? _____

6. Which elbow flexors attach to the humerus?

   _____

7. For each of the motions of the elbow and forearm listed, check the muscle(s) that are the major contributors to the motion.

Motions	Brachialis	Brachioradialis	Biceps Brachii	Supinator	Triceps Brachii	Pronator Teres	Pronator Quadratus
Flexion							
Extension							
Supination							
Pronation							

8. List the joint positions that create passive insufficiency of the

   A. triceps brachii. _____

   B. biceps brachii. _____

9. List the joint positions that create active insufficiency of the

   A. triceps brachii. _____

   B. biceps brachii. _____

10. Identify the following nonmuscular structures:

    A. This structure crosses the elbow vertically on the radial side, attaching to the humerus and ulna.

    _____

    B. This structure crosses the elbow vertically on the ulnar side, attaching to the humerus and ulna.

    _____

    C. This structure attaches only to the ulna.

    _____

    D. This structure connects the ulna and the radius via a broad attachment. _____

11. In the following activities, determine if the distal attachment is moving toward the proximal attachment or if the proximal attachment is moving toward the distal attachment.

12. A person sustained a midshift fracture of the humerus. A complication of this injury was damage to the radial nerve, resulting in muscle paralysis.

    A. Which elbow and/or forearm muscles will have lost innervation?

    _____

    B. What motion(s) will the person have difficulty performing?

    _____

13. Why must a muscle attach on the radius to be able to pronate or supinate the forearm?

    _____

14. When elbow flexion without supination is desired, which muscle(s) prevents supination?

    _____

Activity	Proximal to Distal	Distal to Proximal
An individual pulls on a rope to bring a boat to shore.		
An individual climbs up a rope.		

Which of the above activities is an example of a reversal of muscle action?

_____

Wrist Joint

■ ■ ■ Pre-Lab Worksheets

Student's Name _____

Date Due _____

Complete the following questions prior to the lab class.

1. On Figures 12-1 and 12-2:

A. Label the following joints:

| Radiocarpal joint | Midcarpal joint | Carpometacarpal joint |

B. Label the following bones and landmarks:

Scaphoid	Lunate	Triquetrum
Pisiform	Capitate	Hamate
Trapezium	Trapezoid	Radial styloid process
Radius	Ulna	Articular disk
Metacarpals (1–5)		

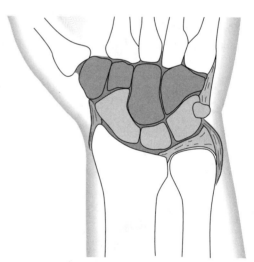

FIGURE 12-2 Bones and landmarks of the wrist.

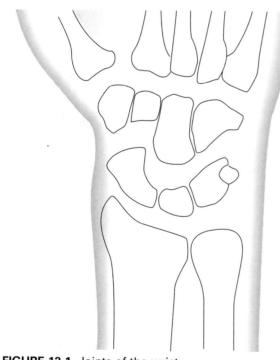

FIGURE 12-1 Joints of the wrist.

2. On Figures 12-3 and 12-4, label the following structures:

Radial collateral ligament   Ulnar collateral ligament

Palmar radiocarpal ligament

3. Draw in the palmar fascia on Figure 12-5.

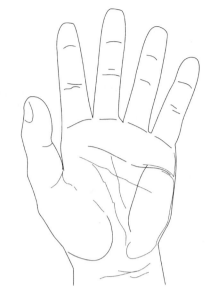

FIGURE 12-5 Palmar fascia.

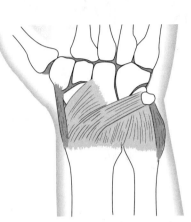

FIGURE 12-3 Ligaments of the wrist, anterior view.

Dorsal radiocarpal ligament   Ulnar styloid process
Radial collateral ligament   Ulnar collateral ligament

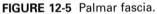

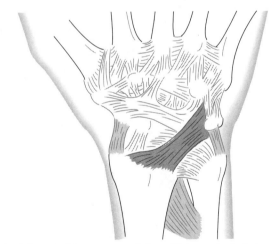

FIGURE 12-4 Ligaments of the wrist, posterior view.

4. On Figures 12-6 and 12-7:

   A. Label the origin and insertion of the muscles shown here. Color the origin in red and the insertion in blue.

   B. Join the origin and insertion to show the direction of the muscle fibers.

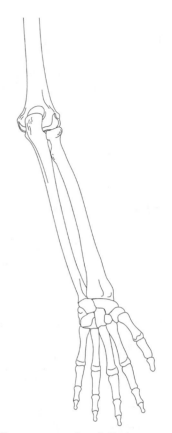

FIGURE 12-7 Extensor carpi radialis longus, extensor carpi radialis brevis, and extensor carpi ulnaris.

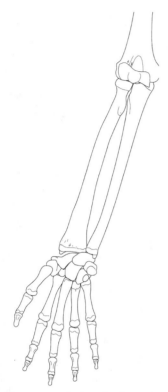

FIGURE 12-6 Flexor carpi ulnaris, flexor carpi radialis, and palmaris longus.

5. Match each function or characteristic with the appropriate structure. Use each term only once.

   _____ Limits extension   A. Radial collateral ligament

   _____ Filler between ulna and adjacent carpals   B. Ulnar collateral ligament

   _____ Provides lateral support   C. Palmar radiocarpal ligament

   _____ Limits flexion   D. Dorsal radiocarpal ligament

   _____ Provides protection and muscle attachment   E. Dorsal radiocarpal ligament

   _____ Provides medial support   F. Articular disk

6. For the following joints, identify the type and
   number of planes of motion available.

Joint	Shape	Degrees of Freedom	Motions	Planes	Axis
Radiocarpal					
Midcarpal					

7. For the radiocarpal joint, identify which surface is
   concave and which is convex.

   Concave: _____

   Convex: _____

8. For the radiocarpal joint, identify the close-packed
   position and the loose-packed positions (refer to
   Chapter 4, Table 4-4).

Joint	Close-Packed	Loose-Packed
Radiocarpal		

9. The end feel of a normal radiocarpal joint (refer to
   Chapter 4 for descriptions)

   Flexion   ____ Bony   ____ Soft tissue stretch   ____ Soft tissue approximation
   Extension   ____ Bony   ____ Soft tissue stretch   ____ Soft tissue approximation
   Radial deviation ____ Bony   ____ Soft tissue stretch   ____ Soft tissue approximation
   Ulnar deviation ____ Bony   ____ Soft tissue stretch   ____ Soft tissue approximation

10. What is the innervation of the extensor muscles of
    the wrist?

    _____

11. List the structure(s) that limit radial deviation:

    _____

12. List the muscles responsible for ulnar deviation:

    _____

    _____

■ ■ ■ Lab Activities

Student's Name _____

Date Due _____

1. Palpation of bones and landmarks, ligaments, and other structures:
   - Locate on bones, skeleton, and your lab partner.
   - The reference position is the anatomical position.
   - Not all structures can be palpated on your partner.

Radius

Styloid process	Projection at the distal end of the radius. Palpate at the distal lateral aspect of the radius. Note that the radial styloid process lies more distal than the ulnar styloid process (see Fig. 11-18).

Ulna

Styloid process	Projection at the distal end of the ulna. Palpate the distal posterior aspect of the ulna. Note that the ulnar styloid process is more prominent than the radial styloid process (see Fig. 11-16).

Proximal Row of Carpal Bones

Scaphoid	Located in the proximal row of carpal bones. Palpate on the radial side of the wrist just distal to the radial styloid process and in line with the thumb.

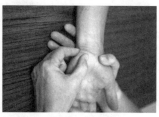

FIGURE 12-8 Palpating the scaphoid.

Lunate	Located in the proximal row of carpal bones in line with the middle finger. Palpate on the dorsal surface by sliding your thumb toward the wrist along the middle metacarpal past the capitate.

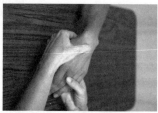

FIGURE 12-9 Palpating the lunate.

Triquetrum	Located in the proximal row of carpal bones on the ulnar side of the wrist just distal to the ulna and in line with the fourth and fifth fingers. The articular disk lies between the ulna and the triquetrum. From palpating the lunate move laterally.
Pisiform	A small bone that appears to lie on the triquetrum on the anterior surface of the wrist inline with the fifth finger. Palpate it on the palmar surface on the ulnar side. The pisiform is more superficial than the hook of the hamate and is often confused with the hook of the hamate.

FIGURE 12-10 Palpating the pisiform.

Distal Row of Carpal Bones

Trapezium	Located in the distal row of carpal bones on the radial side. It articulates with the first metacarpal bone (thumb). Palpate by moving your thumb proximally along the first metacarpal.

Continued

Distal Row of Carpal Bones—cont'd

Trapezoid	A small bone just medial to the trapezium in the distal row of carpal bones. It articulates with the second metacarpal bone. Palpate on the dorsal surface by sliding your thumb toward the wrist along the second metacarpal.
Capitate	The largest carpal bone of the distal row. It articulates with the third metacarpal and part of the fourth metacarpal bones. With the wrist in palmar flexion, palpate the capitate by moving your thumb proximally along the dorsal surface of the metacarpal bone of the middle finger to an indentation just proximal to the third metacarpal. The capitate lies in this indentation. The capitate can be used as the reference point to locate many of the other carpal bones. **FIGURE 12-11** Palpating the capitate.
Hamate	Located on the ulnar side of the wrist medial to the capitate and in line with the fourth and fifth metacarpals. Palpate the hamate by grasping it between your thumb and first finger on the ulnar side of the wrist.
Hook of the hamate	The projection on the palmar surface of the hamate. The hook can be palpated using the tip of your thumb, with deep pressure applied just medial to the longitudinal arches at the wrist. **FIGURE 12-12** Palpating the hook of the hamate.

Other Structures

Radial collateral ligament	Located on the radial side of the wrist. Attachments are the radial styloid process proximally and the scaphoid and trapezium distally. Palpate by placing the pad of one finger over the lateral aspect of the wrist, moving the wrist into ulnar deviation, and feeling the ligament become taut.
Ulnar collateral ligament	Located on the ulnar side of the wrist. Attachments are the ulnar styloid process proximally and the pisiform and triquetrum distally. Palpate by placing the pad of one finger over the medial aspect of the wrist, moving the wrist into radial deviation, and feeling the ligament become taut.
Palmar radiocarpal ligament	Located on the palmar surface of the wrist deep to the wrist and finger tendons. It is a broad, thick band extending from the anterior surface of the distal radius and ulna to the anterior surface of the scaphoid, lunate, and triquetrum. Palpate by placing your finger pads on the lateral aspect of the palmar surface of the wrist and extending the wrist to make the ligament taut. Palpating is difficult because of the many tendons in the area.
Dorsal radiocarpal ligament	Located on the posterior side of the wrist, deep to the wrist and finger extensor tendons. The proximal attachment is on the distal radius, and the distal attachment is the scaphoid, lunate, and triquetrum. This ligament is not as thick as the palmar radiocarpal ligament. Wrist flexion makes the dorsal radiocarpal ligament taut. Palpating is difficult because of the many tendons in the area.
Articular disk	Located on the ulnar side of the wrist between the ulna proximally and the triquetrum distally. Palpate on the ulnar side between the ulna and triquetrum.

Other Structures—cont'd	
Palmar fascia	Also known as the palmar aponeurosis, it is a relatively thick, triangular fascia located superficially at the midline of the palm of the hand. The palmaris longus tendon and the flexor retinaculum blend into this fascia.
Radiocarpal joint	The articulation of the distal radius with the scaphoid and lunate carpal bones. Palpate on the lateral side of the wrist.
Midcarpal joint	The articulation between the proximal and distal rows of carpal bones. Although not a true joint, it is often considered as such. Palpate the individual bones as previously described.

2. Palpation of muscles:

A. Locate the following muscles on the skeleton and anatomical models, and on at least one partner.

- The information needed to palpate each muscle is provided in the following tables.
- The position described for locating the muscle on your partner is usually the manual muscle test position for a fair or better grade of muscle strength.
- Not all origins, insertions, and muscle bellies can be palpated on your partner.

B. On the skeleton, locate the origin and insertion of each muscle.

- Place the ends of a rubber band at the origin and insertion of the muscle, making the band taut. Note the location of the muscle in relation to the joints it crosses.
- When possible, move the skeleton to perform the muscle's motion and observe how the band becomes less taut, similar to the change in length as it performs a concentric contraction.
- Return the skeleton to the starting position and observe how the band becomes taut, similar to the change in length that occurs as it performs an eccentric contraction.

Sitting Position	
FLEXOR CARPI ULNARIS:	Located superficially on the anterior ulnar side of the forearm
	FIGURE 12-13 Palpating the flexor carpi ulnaris.
Position of person:	Sit with the elbow flexed to 90°, the forearm supinated and supported on a table, and the wrist in the neutral position.
Origin:	Medial epicondyle of the humerus
Insertion:	Pisiform, hamate, and base of the fifth metacarpal
Line of pull:	Vertical on the anterior medial surface
Muscle action:	Wrist flexion, ulnar deviation
Palpate:	The tendon on the anterior ulnar side of the wrist, and the muscle belly on the anterior ulnar side of the forearm approximately 2 to 3 inches below the elbow
Instructions to person:	Flex your wrist toward the little finger side while lifting your hand off the table.
FLEXOR CARPI RADIALIS:	Located superficially on the anterior forearm
	FIGURE 12-14 Palpating the flexor carpi radialis.
Position of person:	Sit with the elbow flexed to 90°, the forearm supinated and supported on a table, and the wrist in the neutral position

Continued

Sitting Position—cont'd

Origin:	Medial epicondyle of the humerus
Insertion:	Base of the second and third metacarpal bones
Line of pull:	Vertical on the anterior lateral surface
Muscle action:	Wrist flexion, radial deviation
Palpate:	The tendon on the anterior radial side of the wrist, and the muscle belly on the anterior and slightly medial surface of the forearm just proximal to the midpoint between the medial epicondyle and the carpometacarpal joint of the thumb. When an individual has a palmaris longus muscle, the flexor carpi radialis tendon lies lateral to the palmaris longus tendon.
Instructions to person:	Flex your wrist toward the thumb side while lifting your hand off the table.
PALMARIS LONGUS:	Located superficially in the midline of the anterior forearm

FIGURE 12-15 Palpating the palmaris longus.

Position of person:	Sit with the elbow flexed to 90°, the forearm supinated and supported on a table, and the wrist in the neutral position
Origin:	Medial epicondyle of the humerus
Insertion:	Palmar fascia
Line of pull:	Vertical on the anterior surface
Muscle action:	Assists in wrist flexion
Palpate:	The tendon is in the midline on the anterior surface of the wrist medial to the flexor carpi radialis tendon. This muscle is absent in some individuals bilaterally, and some individuals have only one.

Instructions to person:	Flex your wrist while lifting your hand off the table.
EXTENSOR CARPI RADIALIS LONGUS:	Located superficially on the posterior radial side of the forearm

FIGURE 12-16 Palpating the extensor carpi radialis longus.

Position of person:	Sit with the elbow flexed to 90°, the forearm pronated and supported on a table, and the wrist in the neutral position
Origin:	Supracondylar ridge of the humerus
Insertion:	Base of the second metacarpal bone
Line of pull:	Vertical on the posterior surface
Muscle action:	Wrist extension, radial deviation
Palpate:	The tendon on the dorsal side of the wrist proximal to the insertion on the second metacarpal, and the muscle belly on the lateral aspect of the forearm just distal to the elbow
Instructions to person:	Extend your wrist toward the thumb side by lifting your hand off the table.

Sitting Position—cont'd

EXTENSOR CARPI RADIALIS BREVIS:	Located superficially on the posterior radial side of the forearm

FIGURE 12-17 Palpating the extensor carpi radialis brevis. Note that the examiner's shorter index and longer middle fingers are at the insertions of the extensor carpi radialis brevis (short) and longus (long), respectively.

Position of person:	Sit with the elbow flexed to 90°, the forearm pronated and supported on a table, and the wrist in the neutral position
Origin:	Lateral epicondyle of the humerus
Insertion:	Base of the third metacarpal bone
Line of pull:	Vertical on the posterior surface near the midline
Muscle action:	Wrist extension
Palpate:	The tendon on the dorsal side of the wrist proximal to the insertion on the third metacarpal, and the muscle belly on the lateral aspect posterior side of the proximal forearm. The examiner's middle finger and index finger are on the tendons of the extensor carpi radialis brevis and longus, respectively.
Instructions to person:	Extend your wrist by lifting your hand off the table.

EXTENSOR CARPI ULNARIS:	Located superficially on the posterior radial side of the forearm

FIGURE 12-18 Palpating the extensor carpi ulnaris.

Position of person:	Sit with the elbow flexed to 90°, the forearm pronated and supported on a table, and the wrist in the neutral position
Origin:	Lateral epicondyle of the humerus
Insertion:	Base of the fifth metacarpal
Line of pull:	Diagonally with a large vertical component on the posterior medial surface
Muscle action:	Wrist extension, ulnar deviation
Palpate:	The tendon on the dorsal side of the wrist between the ulnar styloid process and the fifth metacarpal, and the muscle belly on the lateral aspect posterior side of the proximal forearm
Instructions to person:	Extend your wrist toward the little finger side by lifting your hand off the table.

3. Palpate you partner's pulse at the anterior distal lateral aspect of the forearm just proximal to the wrist. What artery are you palpating?

_____

4. Draw the paths of the radial, median, and ulnar nerves as they traverse the forearm and wrist. List the muscles each innervates.

Radial	Median	Ulnar

5. Perform the motions of the wrist with your partner.

   A. Perform a motion and then your partner names the motions you performed.

   B. Your partner names a motion and then you perform that motion.

6. Using the pre-lab worksheets for Question 6 as a reference, for each of the motions available at the following joints:

   A. Place your open left hand in the correct orientation to represent the plane of a motion.

   B. Place your right index finger to indicate the axis of that motion.

   C. Enter the plane and axis for each motion in the following chart.

Radiocarpal Joint	Plane	Axis
Flexion/Extension		
Radial/Ulnar Deviation		
Circumduction		

7. Observe the amount of motion available at the radiocarpal joint in each plane. For each of the motions available at the radiocarpal joint, estimate the degree of motion available by checking the box that *most closely* describes that amount of motion. (Do not measure with a goniometer.)

Motions	0°–45°	46°–90°	91°–135°
Flexion			
Extension			
Radial deviation			
Ulnar deviation			

8. Move your partner's wrist passively through the available range of motion making note of the end feel. If possible, repeat with several people. Review question 9 in the worksheets for normal end feel.

   A. Is your partner's end feel consistent with normal end feel for the following?

   _____ Flexion/extension

   _____ Radial/ulnar deviation

   B. Name the structures that create the end feel for the following motions:

   Flexion: _____

   Extension: _____

   Radial deviation: _____

   Ulnar deviation: _____

9. Use a disarticulated skeleton or anatomical model of the radiocarpal joint and apply the rules of joint arthrokinematics and the concave-convex rule to perform the following activities:

   A. Underline the correct answer.
      The radius is concave/convex.
      The carpals are concave/convex.

   B. Observe the movement of the proximal row of carpal bones on the radius. Circle the motions that you observed.

   Roll   Spin   Glide

10. Analyze opening a jar:

   A. Using your *right hand,* open a jar with a screw-on lid. Does your hand move into radial or ulnar deviation as you loosen the lid?

   _____

   B. Replace the lid on the jar using your *right hand.* Does your hand move into radial or ulnar deviation as you tighten the lid?

   _____

   C. Using your *left hand,* open a jar with a screw-on lid. Does your hand move into radial or ulnar deviation as you loosen the lid?

   _____

   D. Replace the lid on the jar using your *left hand.* Does your hand move into radial or ulnar deviation as you tighten the lid?

   _____

11. **Functional activity analysis:**

In each chapter on the upper extremity you will analyze the activity of placing a plate in a cabinet then removing the plate and placing it on the counter. Perform those tasks and then analyze how the subject in Figures 12-19 and 12-20 performed those tasks.

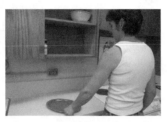

FIGURE 12-19 Starting position of placing plate in cabinet.

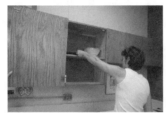

FIGURE 12-20 Starting position of placing a plate on counter.

A. Describe the positions of the wrist when the subject is

 1) starting to remove the plate from the cabinet shelf. _____

 2) placing the plate on the counter. _____

B. Which wrist muscle groups are acting as

 1) the plate is being lowered from the cabinet shelf to the counter? _____

 2) the plate is being raised from the counter to the cabinet shelf? _____

C. Describe the type of muscle contraction being used and why as

 1) the plate is being lowered from the cabinet shelf to the counter.

 _____

 2) the plate is being raised from the counter to the cabinet shelf.

 _____

■ ■ ■ Post-Lab Questions

Student's Name _____

Date Due _____

After you have completed the worksheets and lab activities, answer the following questions without using your book or notes. When finished, check your answers.

1. The wrist flexors share a common proximal attachment on or in the area of the:

   _____

2. List the muscles of the wrist that attach on the posterior side of the wrist.

   _____

3. List the two muscles that attach on the base of the fifth metacarpal.

   _____

4. Which muscle does not have two bony attachments, and what is its nonbony attachment?

   _____

5. List the muscles that act together to produce ulnar deviation of the wrist.

   _____

6. When the muscles listed in the following table perform the movement listed, identify the movement that must be neutralized and list the neutralizing muscles.

Movement and Muscle	Movement to Be Neutralized	Neutralizing Muscles
Wrist extension by extensor carpi radialis longus		
Wrist flexion by flexor carpi ulnaris		

7. Can the position of the elbow joint affect the range of motion of the wrist? _____

Explain your answer. _____

_____

_____

8. Explain why the extensor carpi radialis brevis does not play a major role in wrist radial deviation.

   _____

9. An individual with a diagnosis of ulnar nerve entrapment has signs of muscle weakness. Which wrist muscle(s) would be involved?

   _____

10. Loss of radial nerve function results in a condition known as "wrist drop." Explain why.

    _____

    _____

11. Starting on the anterior medial side and proceeding laterally around the wrist, name the wrist muscles in the order encountered.

    _____

    _____

12. The wrist flexors and extensors are generally innervated by which nerves?

    A. Wrist extensors: _____

    B. Wrist flexors: _____

    C. List the exception(s): _____

13. In the photograph shown here, which of the person's wrists does not have a palmaris longus muscle tendon?

    _____ Right _____ Left

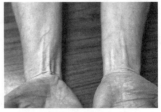

FIGURE 12-21 Palmaris longus.

Hand

■ ■ ■ **Pre-Lab Worksheets**

Student's Name _____

Date Due _____

Complete the following questions prior to the lab class.

1. A. What is the distinction between intrinsic and extrinsic muscles?

_____

_____

B. What is another word for prehension?

_____

C. List the types of prehension.

_____

_____

2. Label the structures on Figures 13-1 through 13-4 using the names given:

A. Label the joints and bones:

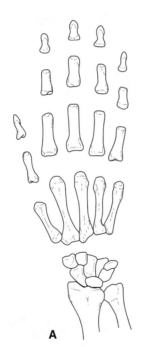

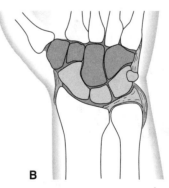

A   **B**

FIGURE 13-1 (A) Joints and bones of the hand and wrist. **(B)** Bones of the wrist.

Carpometacarpal joints (CMC)	Metacarpophalangeal joints (MCP)	Lunate	Pisiform
Interphalangeal joints (DIP, PIP, IP)	Metacarpals 1–5	Hamate	Trapezium
Phalanges: proximal, middle, distal	Scaphoid	Trapezoid	Capitate
		Triquetrum	

B. On Figure 13-2, label the following structures:

Flexor retinaculum   Palmar carpal ligament

Transverse carpal
    ligament

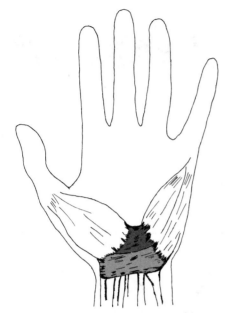

FIGURE 13-2 Flexor retinaculum.

C. On Figure 13-3, draw in the extensor
retinaculum.

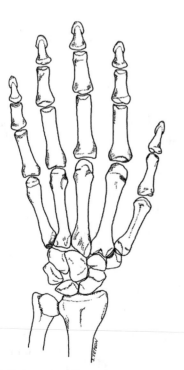

FIGURE 13-3 Extensor retinaculum.

D. Label the following arches on Figure 13-4:

Proximal carpal arch   Distal carpal arch

Longitudinal arch

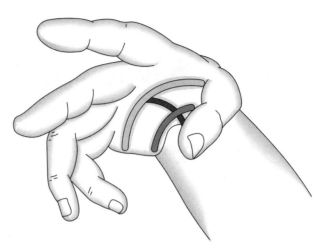

FIGURE 13-4. Arches of hand.

3. On Figures 13-5 through 13-11:

A. Label the origin and insertion of the muscles listed.
Color the origin in red and the insertion in blue.

B. Join the origin and insertion to show the line
of pull.

FIGURE 13-5 Flexor digitorum superficialis, flexor
digitorum profundus, and flexor pollicis longus.

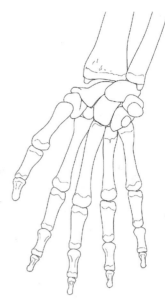

FIGURE 13-8 Opponens digiti minimi, flexor digiti minimi, and abductor digiti minimi.

FIGURE 13-6 Extensor digitorum, extensor digiti minimi, extensor indicis, abductor pollicis longus, extensor pollicis longus, and extensor pollicis brevis.

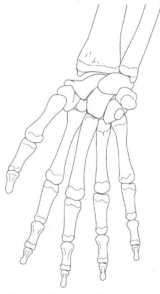

FIGURE 13-9 Palmar interossei.

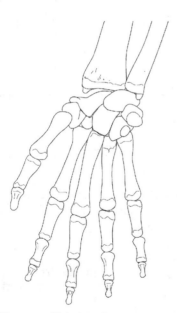

FIGURE 13-7 Flexor pollicis brevis, opponens pollicis, abductor pollicis brevis, and adductor pollicis.

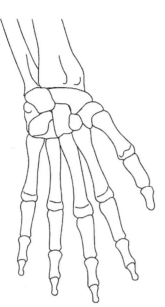

FIGURE 13-10 Dorsal interossei.

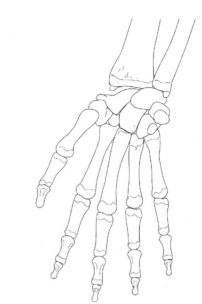

FIGURE 13-11 Lumbricales.

4. For each joint listed, identify the following:

Joint	Shape	Degrees of Freedom	Motions	Plane	Axis
Thumb CMC					
Thumb MP					
Thumb IP					
Finger MP					
Finger PIP					
Finger DIP					

5. At each of the joints, identify which surface is concave and which is convex.

Joint	Concave	Convex
Finger DIP and PIP		
Metacarpophalangeal		
Thumb CMC		
Thumb IP		

6. For each of the following finger joints, provide the close-packed position and the loose-packed position (refer to Chapter 4, Table 4-4 for descriptions).

Joint	Close-Packed	Loose-Packed
DIP and PIP		
Metacarpophalangeal		

7. For each of the following finger joints, describe the end feel (refer to Chapter 4 for descriptions).

Joint	End Feel
DIP and PIP	
Metacarpophalangeal	

8. The tendons of which muscles pass through the carpal tunnel?

_____

_____

_____

9. Which nerve passes through the carpal tunnel?

_____

_____

10. For each muscle listed in the following table, check the motions for which the muscle is considered a prime mover for motions of the thumb or fingers.

Muscle	Flexion	Extension	Abduction	Adduction	Opposition
Flexor digitorum superficialis					
Flexor digitorum profundus					
Extensor digitorum					
Extensor digiti minimi					
Extensor indicis					
Abductor pollicis longus					
Extensor pollicis longus					
Extensor pollicis brevis					
Flexor pollicis longus					
Flexor pollicis brevis					
Abductor pollicis brevis					
Opponens pollicis					
Adductor pollicis					
Flexor digiti minimi					
Abductor digiti minimi					
Opponens digiti minimi					
Dorsal interossei					
Palmar interossei					
Lumbricales					

11. Match the following ligament and structure with the appropriate function or characteristic. Each term may be used more than once. Each function or characteristic may have more than one answer.

_____ Is located on the anterior surface   A. Flexor retinaculum

_____ Composed retinaculum of two parts   B. Extensor

_____ Is part of the carpal tunnel   C. Extensor expansion

_____ Holds tendons close to wrist   D. Transverse carpal ligament

_____ Is located on the posterior surface   E. Palmar carpal ligament

_____ Is located on the posterior and sides of the proximal phalanges

_____ Provides attachment of extensor tendons to middle and distal phalanges

12. Of the extrinsic muscles of the hand, identify which joints each muscle crosses by placing in the cell the position that lengthens the muscle over that joint.

Muscle	Elbow	Wrist	CMC	MP	PIP	DIP	Thumb IP
Flexor digitorum superficialis							
Flexor digitorum profundus							
Flexor pollicis longus							
Extensor digitorum							
Extensor digiti minimi							
Extensor indicis							
Abductor pollicis longus							
Extensor pollicis longus							
Extensor pollicis brevis							

■ ■ ■ Lab Activities

Student's Name _____

Date Due _____

1. Palpation of bones and landmarks, ligaments, and other structures:
   - Locate on bones, skeleton, and your lab partner.
   - The reference position is the anatomical position.
   - Not all structures can be palpated on your partner.

Thumb

First metacarpal	Palpate by grasping the thumb just above the carpometacarpal joint. Articulates with the trapezium bone and proximal phalange. 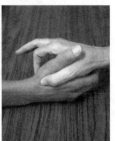 **FIGURE 13-12** Palpating first metacarpal.
Proximal phalange	Palpate by grasping the thumb just above the metacarpophalangeal joint. Articulates with the first metacarpal bone and the distal phalange.
Distal phalange	Palpate by grasping the end of the thumb. Articulates with the proximal phalange.
Carpometacarpal joint (CMC)	Palpate the CMC joint on the palmar radial side of the hand at the wrist. The trapezium articulates with the base of the metacarpal. 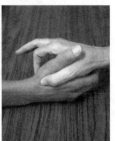 **FIGURE 13-13** Palpating thumb CMC.
Metacarpophalangeal joint (MP)	Palpate the MP joint at the distal end of the metacarpal as it articulates with the proximal phalange.
Interphalangeal joint (IP)	Palpate the IP joint at the junction of the proximal and distal phalanges.

Fingers: Digits 2–5

Metacarpals	Palpate on the dorsum of the hand. The long bones of the hand lie between the wrist and the fingers. The bases of the metacarpals articulate with the distal row of the carpal bones. The heads of the metacarpals articulate with the proximal phalanges of the fingers. 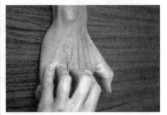 **FIGURE 13-14** Palpating the metacarpals.

Continued

Fingers: Digits 2–5—Cont'd

Proximal phalange	Palpate by grasping a finger just distal to the MP joints of the fingers.
Middle phalange	Palpate by grasping a finger between the IP joints.
Distal phalange	Palpate by grasping the end of a finger distal to the DIP joint.
Carpometacarpal joint (CMC)	Palpate on the dorsum of the hand by moving proximally on the metacarpals. This is the articulation of the distal row of carpal bones with the metacarpals. **FIGURE 13-15** Palpating the CMC.
Metacarpophalangeal joint (MP)	Also called "knuckles," these joints are palpated by grasping the metacarpal with one hand and the adjunct proximal phalange with the other hand. Move the phalange on the metacarpal noting where the motion occurs. Move the hand from the metacarpal to the area where the motion is occurring.
Proximal interphalangeal joint (PIP)	Palpate by stabilizing the proximal phalange with one hand and grasping the middle phalange with the other hand. Move the middle phalange on the proximal phalange, noting where the motion occurs. Move the hand from the proximal phalange to the area where the motion is occurring.
Distal interphalangeal joint (DIP)	Palpate by stabilizing the middle phalange with one hand and grasping the distal phalange with the other hand. Move the distal phalange on the middle phalange, noting where the motion occurs. Move the hand from the middle phalange to the area where the motion is occurring.

2. Palpation of muscles:

A. Locate the following muscles on the skeleton and anatomical models, and on at least one partner.

- The information needed to palpate each muscle is provided in the following tables.
- The position described for locating the muscle on your partner is usually the manual muscle test position for a fair or better grade of muscle strength.
- Not all origins, insertions, and muscle bellies can be palpated on your partner.

B. On the skeleton, locate the origin and insertion of each muscle.

- Place the ends of a rubber band at the origin and insertion of the muscle, making the band taut. Note the location of the muscle in relation to the joints it crosses.
- When possible, move the skeleton to perform the muscle's motion and observe how the band becomes less taut, similar to the change in length as it performs a concentric contraction.
- Return the skeleton to the starting position and observe how the band becomes taut, similar to the change in length as it performs an eccentric contraction.

Sitting Position With the Elbow Flexed to 90° and the Forearm Supported on a Table

FLEXOR DIGITORUM SUPERFICIALIS:	On the anterior surface, located deep to the wrist flexors and the palmaris longus
Position of person:	Forearm supinated, and wrist and fingers in neutral position
Origin:	Common flexor tendon on the medial epicondyle of the humerus, coronoid process, and radius
Insertion:	Each side of the middle phalange of the four fingers
Line of pull:	Vertical on the anterior surface
Muscle action:	Flexes the MCP and PIP joints of the fingers

Palpate:	The tendon at the wrist lateral and deep to the palmaris longus, and the muscle belly on the anterior surface of the forearm distal to the elbow
Instructions to person:	Bend the first two joints of your fingers so that the pads of the fingers rest against your palm.
FLEXOR DIGITORUM PROFUNDUS:	Located deep to the flexor digitorum superficialis on the anterior surface of the forearm and hand
Position of person:	Forearm supinated, and wrist and fingers in neutral
Origin:	Upper three-fourths of the ulna
Insertion:	Distal phalange of the four fingers
Line of pull:	Mostly vertical on the anterior surface
Muscle action:	Flexes MCP, PIP, and DIP joints of the fingers
Palpate:	Difficult to palpate the tendon because it is deep to other tendons, and the muscle belly is on the anterior surface of the forearm distal to the elbow.
Instructions to person:	Curl your fingers into your palm.
EXTENSOR DIGITORUM:	Located superficially on the posterior forearm and hand.

FIGURE 13-16 Palpating the extensor digitorum tendons.

Position of person:	Forearm pronated, and wrist and fingers in neutral
Origin:	Lateral epicondyle of the humerus

Insertion:	Base of the distal phalange of fingers 2–5
Line of pull:	Mostly vertical on the posterior surface
Muscle action:	Extends the MCP, PIP, and DIP joints of the fingers
Palpate:	The tendons can be palpated on the dorsum of the hand, and the muscle bellies are palpated on the proximal posterior lateral forearm.
Instructions to person:	Straighten and lift your fingers off the table.
EXTENSOR DIGITI MINIMI:	Located deep to the extensor digitorum and extensor carpi ulnaris muscles at its origin. Located superficially on the posterior medial surface of the wrist.
Position of person:	Forearm pronated, and wrist and fifth finger in neutral
Origin:	Lateral epicondyle of the humerus
Insertion:	Base of the distal phalange of the fifth finger
Line of pull:	Mostly vertical on the posterior surface
Muscle action:	Extends the MCP, PIP, and DIP joints of the fifth finger
Palpate:	On the dorsum of the hand over the fifth metacarpal lateral to the extensor digitorum
Instructions to person:	Straighten and lift your little finger.
EXTENSOR INDICIS:	Located deep on the posterior lateral surface of the forearm
Position of person:	Forearm pronated and wrist and index finger in neutral
Origin:	Posterior surface of distal ulna
Insertion:	The extensor hood at the base of the distal phalange

Continued

Sitting Position With the Elbow Flexed to 90° and the Forearm Supported on a Table—Cont'd

Line of pull:	Mostly vertical on the posterior surface
Muscle action:	Extends the MCP, PIP, and DIP joints of the index finger
Palpate:	The tendon on the dorsum of the hand over the second metacarpal medial to the tendon of the extensor digitorum, and the muscle belly on the posterior distal ulna
Instructions to person:	Straighten and lift your index finger off the table.
FLEXOR POLLICIS LONGUS:	Located deep on the anterior surface of the forearm
Position of person:	Forearm supinated, and the wrist in neutral, the thumb resting on the palm over the second metacarpal
Origin:	Anterior surface of the radius
Insertion:	Distal phalange of the thumb
Line of pull:	Mostly vertical
Muscle action:	Flexes the CMC, MCP, and IP joints of the thumb
Palpate:	The tendon on the palmar surface of the proximal phalange, and the muscle belly on the anterior surface of the radius about two-thirds of distance from the elbow
Instructions to person:	Curl your thumb into your palm.
ABDUCTOR POLLICIS LONGUS:	Located deep on the posterior forearm

FIGURE 13-17 Palpating the abductor pollicis longus.

Position of person:	Forearm in mid position and wrist in neutral, thumb in resting position
Origin:	Posterior surface of the radius, interosseous membrane, and posterior lateral surface of the middle portion of the ulna
Insertion:	Radial side of the base of the first metacarpal
Line of pull:	Mostly vertical
Muscle action:	Abducts the thumb
Palpate:	The tendon at the insertion. This tendon lies next to the extensor pollicis brevis tendon to make up the lateral border of the anatomical snuffbox.
Instructions to person:	Move your thumb toward ceiling.
EXTENSOR POLLICIS LONGUS:	Located deep on the posterior forearm
Position of person:	Forearm in midposition, wrist and thumb in neutral
Origin:	Posterior lateral side of the ulna and the interosseous membrane
Insertion:	Base of the distal phalange of the thumb
Line of pull:	Vertical
Muscle action:	Extends the CMC, MCP, and IP joints of the thumb
Palpate:	The tendon on the dorsum of the proximal phalange. The extensor pollicis longus tendon is on the index finger side of the anatomical snuffbox.
Instructions to person:	Move your thumb out to the side.
EXTENSOR POLLICIS BREVIS:	Located deep on the posterior distal forearm
Position of person:	Forearm in midposition and the wrist in neutral
Origin:	Posterior distal surface of the radius

Insertion:	Base of the proximal phalange of the thumb		Muscle action:	Abducts the thumb
Line of pull:	Mostly vertical		Palpate:	The muscle belly in the thenar group on the lateral side of the first metacarpal
Muscle action:	Extends the CMC and MCP joints of the thumb		Instructions to person:	Lift your thumb off your palm.
Palpate:	The tendon at the insertion. This tendon is on the thumb side of the anatomical snuffbox.		***OPPONENS POLLICIS:***	Located deep in the palm
Instructions to person:	Move your thumb out to the side.			FIGURE 13-18 Palpating the opponens pollicis.
FLEXOR POLLICIS BREVIS:	Located superficially in the thenar group			
Position of person:	Forearm supinated, and the wrist and thumb in neutral		Position of person:	Forearm supinated, and the wrist and thumb in neutral
Origin:	Trapezium, trapezoid, capitate, and flexor retinaculum		Origin:	Trapezium and flexor retinaculum
Insertion:	Base of the proximal phalange of the thumb		Insertion:	First metacarpal
Line of pull:	Vertical		Line of pull:	Diagonal and wrapping around the bone, making it spiral
Muscle action:	Flexes the CMC and MCP joints while maintaining the IP joint extended		Muscle action:	Opposes the thumb and little finger by touching the pad of the thumb to the pad of the little finger
Palpate:	The muscle belly in the middle of the thenar group proximal to the metacarpophalangeal joint		Palpate:	On the radial side of the first metacarpal, lateral to the abductor pollicis brevis
Instructions to person:	Bend your thumb into your palm, keeping the last joint of your thumb straight.		Instructions to person:	Touch the pad of your thumb to the pad of your little finger.
ABDUCTOR POLLICIS BREVIS:	Located superficially in the thenar group		***ADDUCTOR POLLICIS:***	Located deep in the palm
Position of person:	Forearm supinated, the wrist in neutral, and thumb resting on the palmar surface of the second metacarpal.			FIGURE 13-19 Palpating the adductor pollicis.
Origin:	Scaphoid, trapezium, and the flexor retinaculum			
Insertion:	Radial side of the base of the proximal phalanx of the thumb		Position of person:	Forearm pronated with the hand off the edge of the table, the wrist in neutral, and the thumb in abduction
Line of pull:	Vertical			

Continued

Sitting Position With the Elbow Flexed to 90° and the Forearm Supported on a Table—Cont'd

Origin:	Capitate, base of the second metacarpal, and palmar surface of the metacarpal
Insertion:	Base of the proximal phalange of the thumb
Line of pull:	Horizontal
Muscle action:	Adducts the thumb by bringing it toward the palm
Palpate:	In the web space between the first and second metacarpals
Instructions to person:	Move your thumb into your palm.
FLEXOR DIGITI MINIMI:	Located in the hypothenar group
Position of person:	Forearm supinated, and the wrist and fifth finger in neutral
Origin:	Hamate and flexor retinaculum
Insertion:	Base of the proximal phalange of the fifth finger
Line of pull:	Vertical
Muscle action:	Flexes the CMC and MCP joints of the fifth finger
Palpate:	In the hypothenar eminence on the anterior surface over the distal end of the fifth metacarpal
Instructions to person:	Curl your little finger into your palm.
ABDUCTOR DIGITI MINIMI:	Located superficially on the ulnar border of the hypothenar eminence

FIGURE 13-20 Palpating the abductor digiti minimi.

Position of person:	Forearm supinated, and wrist and fifth finger in neutral

Origin:	Pisiform and tendon of the flexor carpi ulnaris
Insertion:	Medial side of the base of the proximal phalange of the fifth finger
Line of pull:	Vertical
Muscle action:	Abducts the fifth finger
Palpate:	The muscle belly on the medial aspect of the fifth finger
Instructions to person:	Move your little finger out to the side.
OPPONENS DIGITI MINIMI:	Located deep to the other hypothenar muscles
Position of person:	Forearm supinated, and the wrist and fifth finger in neutral
Origin:	Hamate and flexor retinaculum
Insertion:	Medial side of the fifth metacarpal
Line of pull:	Diagonal and wrapping around the bone, making it spiral
Muscle action:	Opposes the fifth finger by touching the pad of the fifth finger to the pad of the thumb
Palpate:	In the hypothenar eminence on the anterior surface over the proximal end of the fifth metacarpal
Instructions to person:	Touch the pad of your little finger to the pad of your thumb.
DORSAL INTEROSSEI (DI):	Located deep on the dorsum of the hand

FIGURE 13-21 Palpating over the area of the muscle bellies of the dorsal interossei.

Position of person:	Forearm pronated, and the wrist and fingers in neutral.

Origin:	First DI: First and second metacarpals Second DI: Second and third metacarpals Third DI: Third and fourth metacarpals Fourth DI: Fourth and fifth metacarpals
Insertion:	First DI: Lateral side of proximal phalange of index finger Second DI: Lateral side of proximal phalange of middle finger Third DI: Medial side of proximal phalange of middle finger Fourth DI: Medial side of proximal phalange of ring finger
Line of pull:	Vertical
Muscle action:	First DI: Abducts index finger Second DI: Abducts middle finger laterally Third DI: Abducts middle finger medially Fourth DI Abducts ring finger
Palpate:	First DI: At the base of the proximal phalange of the index finger; the remaining dorsal interossei cannot be palpated.
Instructions to person:	Spread your fingers apart.
PALMAR INTEROSSEI (PI):	Located deep in the palm
Position of person:	Forearm supinated, and the wrist and fingers in neutral
Origin:	First PI: First metacarpal Second PI: Second metacarpal Third PI: Fourth metacarpal Fourth PI: Fifth metacarpal
Insertion:	First PI: Medial side of proximal phalange of thumb Second PI: Medial side of proximal phalange of index finger Third PI: Lateral side of proximal phalange of ring finger Fourth PI: Lateral side of proximal phalange of fifth finger

Line of pull:	Vertical
Muscle action:	First PI: Adducts thumb Second PI: Adducts the index finger Third PI: Adducts the ring finger Fourth PI: Adducts the fifth finger
Palpate:	These muscles cannot be palpated.
Instructions to person:	Squeeze your fingers together.
LUMBRICALES	Located deep on the lateral sides of the MP joints
Position of person:	Forearm supinated, wrist and fingers in neutral
Origin:	Tendons of the flexor digitorum profundus muscle
Insertion:	Radial side of the corresponding digit's extensor hood
Line of pull:	Vertical
Muscle action:	Flexes the MP joints and simultaneously extends the IP joints
Palpate:	These small deep muscles cannot be palpated.
Instructions to person:	Starting from a hook grasp position, move your fingers in the opposite directions—bend at the first joint and straighten the other joints.

3. Perform the motions of the thumb and finger joints with your partner.

   A. Perform a motion and have your partner name the motion you performed and the plane of motion.

   B. Your partner names a motion and then you perform that motion.

4. Observe the amount of motion available at each joint in each plane. For each of the motions available at the joints listed in the following tables, estimate the degrees of motion available by checking the box that *most closely* describes that amount of motion. (Do not measure with a goniometer.)

Thumb Carpometacarpal

Motions	0°–45°	46°–90°	91°–135°	136°–180°
Flexion				
Extension				
Abduction				
Adduction				
Opposition				

Thumb Metacarpophalangeal

Motions	0°–45°	46°–90°	91°–135°	136°–180°
Flexion				
Extension				

Finger Metacarpophalangeal

Motions	0°–45°	46°–90°	91°–135°	136°–180°
Flexion				
Extension				
Abduction				
Adduction				

Finger Interphalangeal

Motions	0°–45°	46°–90°	91°–135°	136°–180°
PIP Flexion				
DIP Flexion				

5. Passively move your partner through the available range of motion of the finger IP and MP joints, noting the end feel. If possible, repeat with several people. Review worksheet Question 7 for normal end feel.

   A. Is your partner's end feel consistent with normal end feel?

   B. What structures create normal end feel for the finger?

   MP joint: _____

   IP joint: _____

6. Referring to worksheet Question 12, assume the positions that lengthen the extrinsic hand muscle simultaneously over the joints they cross.

7. Use a disarticulated skeleton or anatomical model of the following joints and apply the rules of joint arthrokinematics and the concave-convex rule to perform the following activities.

   A. **Thumb carpometacarpal joint**

      1) Underline the correct answer.

         The trapezium is concave/convex.

         The metacarpal is concave/convex.

      2) Move the metacarpal on the trapezium in all planes of motion permitted by the joint.

      3) What arthrokinematic motions occur when the metacarpal moves on the trapezium?

         Roll   Spin   Glide

   B. **Thumb and finger metacarpophalangeal joints**

      1) Underline the correct answer.

         The metacarpal is concave/convex.

         The phalange is concave/convex.

      2) Move the proximal phalange on the metacarpal in all planes of motion permitted by the joint.

      3) What arthrokinematic motions occur when the proximal phalange moves on the metacarpal?

         Roll   Spin   Glide

C. **Finger interphalangeal joints**

　1) Underline the correct answer.

　　The distal proximal phalange is concave/convex.

　　The proximal middle phalange is concave/convex.

　2) Move the middle phalanx on the proximal phalanx in all planes of motion permitted by the joint.

　3) What arthrokinematic motions occur when the middle phalange moves on the proximal phalange?

　　Roll　　　　　Spin　　　　　Glide

8. Note the amount of wrist motion in each of the following activities:

　A. With fingers flexed, extend the wrist; then with fingers extended, extend the wrist.

　　Which position of the fingers permitted more wrist extension? _____

　　Why? _____

　　_____

　B. With the fingers extended, flex the wrist. Next, flex the wrist with fingers flexed.

　　Which position of the fingers permitted more wrist flexion? _____

　　Why? _____

　C. How can you determine if active insufficiency or passive insufficiency limits the range of motion?

　　_____

　　_____

9. Perform each of the following types of grasp. Describe one functional task performed with each type of grasp. Do not use the examples from the book.

Power Grips

Grip	Description	Example
Cylindrical	All the fingers flex around an object that usually lies at a right angle to the forearm.	
Spherical	All the fingers and thumb are abducted and then flexed around an object.	
Hook	The IP joints of the fingers are flexed and the thumb does not participate.	

Precision Grips

Grip	Description	Example
Pad-to-pad	Pad of thumb is touched to pad of a finger; MCP and PIP joints of the fingers are flexed; thumb is adducted and the distal IP joints of both are extended.	
Pinch	A pad-to-pad grip involving the thumb and usually the index finger	
Three jaw chuck	Pad-to-pad grip involving the thumb and the index and middle fingers	

Continued

Precision Grips—Cont'd

Grip	Description	Example
Tip-to-tip or pincer	Tip of the thumb is touched against the tip of another digit.	
Pad-to-side or lateral prehension	Pad of the extended thumb presses an object against the radial side of the index finger.	
Side-to-side	Two adjacent fingers are adducted.	
Lumbrical or plate	MCP joints flex and the PIP and DIP joints extend; thumb opposes the fingers.	

10. Describe the conditions that permit the extensor muscles of the wrist to produce grasp.

    _____

    This tendon action of a muscle is also known as:

    _____

11. Hold a piece of paper between your index and middle fingers (or any two adjacent fingers) while your classmate tries to pull the paper out from between your fingers.

    A. Could the paper be removed easily?

       _____

    B. Which muscles were at work and what were their actions?

       _____

    C. Damage to which nerve weakens these muscles?

       _____

12. Functional activity analysis

    In each chapter on the upper extremity you will be analyzing the activity of placing a plate in a cabinet then removing the plate and placing it on the counter. Perform those tasks and then analyze how the subject in Figures 13-22 and 13-23 performed those tasks.

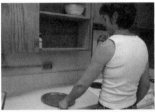

FIGURE 13-22 Starting position of placing plate in cabinet.

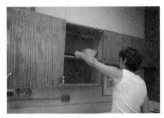

FIGURE 13-23 Starting position of placing plate on counter.

    A. Describe the type of grasp used when the subject holds the plate:

       _____

    B. Which muscle group(s) are maintaining the grasp as the plate is being lowered from the cabinet shelf to the counter?

       _____

    C. Describe the type of muscle contraction being used and why as the plate is being lowered from the cabinet shelf to the counter.

       _____

    D. Does the type of grasp change during the motion of moving the plate from the shelf to the counter and back to the shelf? _____

■ ■ ■ **Post-Lab Questions**

Student's Name _____

Date Due _____

After you have completed the worksheets and lab activities, answer the following questions without using your book or notes. When finished, check your answers.

1. Identify the following muscles according to their location in relation to each other:

   A. What is the most superficial muscle on the anterior surface of the wrist located in the midline of the wrist?

   _____

   B. What muscle or tendon lies directly underneath the muscle identified in A?

   _____

   C. What muscle or tendon lies directly underneath the muscle identified in B?

   _____

2. Are the thenar and hypothenar muscles intrinsic or extrinsic muscles?

   _____

3. Which muscle attaches to the tendons of the flexor digitorum profundus and extensor digitorum muscles?

   _____

4. Thenar muscles control the _____.
   The muscles of the thenar muscle group are the

   _____
   _____.

   These muscles are innervated by the _____ nerve. Damage to this nerve would mean loss of the thumb motions of _____.

5. If one were to generalize about the innervation of the muscles of the hand by their location, the muscles on the

   A. posterior surface are innervated by the

   _____.

   B. anterior medial surface are innervated by the

   _____.

   C. anterior lateral surface are innervated by the

   _____.

6. Which muscles have the combined action of MP flexion and IP extension?

   _____

7. What is the reference point for MP abduction and adduction of the fingers?

   _____

8. The extrinsic muscles involved in finger extension are:

   _____

   _____

   The extrinsic muscles involved in finger flexion are:

   _____

   _____

9. Name the muscle that abducts the index finger:

   _____

   _____

10. Identify the muscle tendons that make up the anatomical snuffbox illustrated in Figure 13-24.

_____

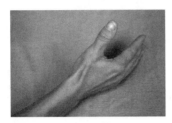

FIGURE 13-24 Anatomical snuffbox.

11. For each of the following grasps, identify the type of grasp and determine if it is a power or precision grasp.

   Picking up a weight bar: _____

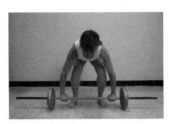

FIGURE 13-25 Picking up a weight bar.

   Grasping a foot: _____

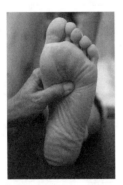

FIGURE 13-26 Grasping a foot.

12. The muscle bellies of many muscles controlling the hand are extrinsic to the hand—being located in the forearm.

   A. Which finger muscle is attached at the medial epicondyle of the humerus?

   _____

   B. Which muscles make up the superficial group of muscles that flex the wrist and fingers?

   _____

   _____

   C. Which finger muscles are attached to the lateral epicondyle?

   _____

13. Which dermatome is responsible for the sensations in the following activities?

   A. Scratching the posterior surface of your fifth finger. _____

   B. Squeezing your thumb. _____

   C. Pinching the palm of your hand near your index finger. _____

Clinical Kinesiology and Anatomy of the Trunk

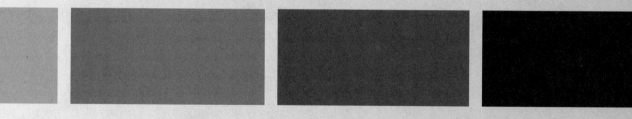

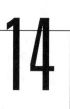
Temporomandibular Joint

■ ■ ■ Pre-Lab Worksheets

Student's Name _____

Date Due _____

Complete the following questions prior to the lab class.

1. Define the following terms:

   Protrusion: _____

   Retrusion or retraction: _____

   Lateral deviation: _____

2. On Figures 14-1 through 14-4, label the following bones and landmarks:

MANDIBLE: Angle   Body   Condyle   Coronoid process

   Neck   Notch   Ramus

LANDMARKS: Articular   Articular   Postglenoid
            tubercle   fossa   tubercle

   Styloid   Mastoid   External
   process   process   auditory
                          meatus

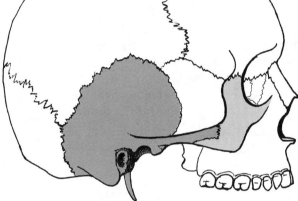

FIGURE 14-2 Landmarks related to the TMJ.

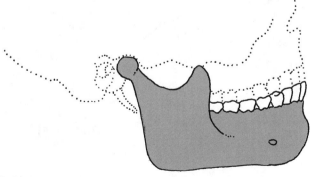

FIGURE 14-1 Mandible, right lateral view.

SPHENOID: Greater wing Lateral pterygoid
of sphenoid plate of sphenoid

MAXILLA: Maxillary
tuberosity

3. On Figure 14-5, shade in the temporal fossa and label the bones that make up the fossa.

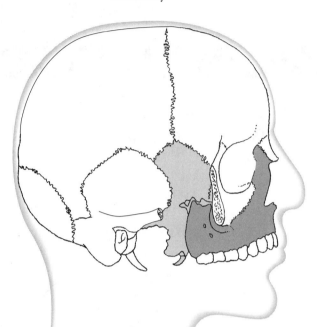

FIGURE 14-3 Lateral view of skull with mandible and zygomatic bones removed.

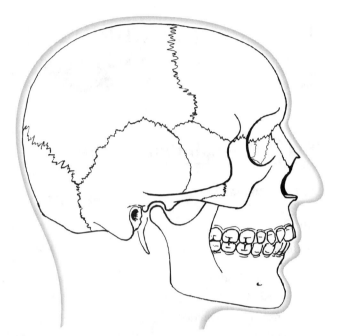

FIGURE 14-5 Lateral view of skull.

| Temporomandibular joint | Hyoid bone | Thyroid cartilage | Epiglottis |
| First cricoid ring | Trachea | Stylohyoid ligament | Styloid process |

4. On Figure 14-6, label the following structures:

Lateral ligament
(temporomandibular ligament)
Sphenomandibular ligament

Stylomandibular ligament
Joint capsule

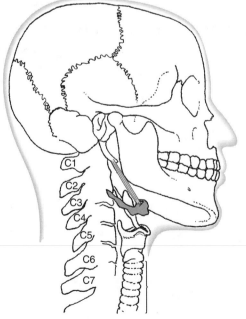

FIGURE 14-4 Lateral view of skull, vertebral column, and trachea.

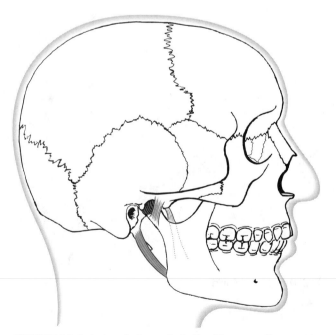

FIGURE 14-6 Lateral view of skull with some ligaments.

5. On Figure 14-7:

   A. Label the origin and insertion of the muscles listed.

   B. Join the origin and insertion to show the line of pull.

   Temporalis   Masseter

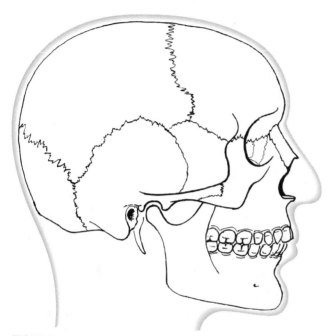

FIGURE 14-7 Lateral view of skull.

6. Identify the medial and lateral pterygoid muscles in Figure 14-8 and label the origin and insertion of each.

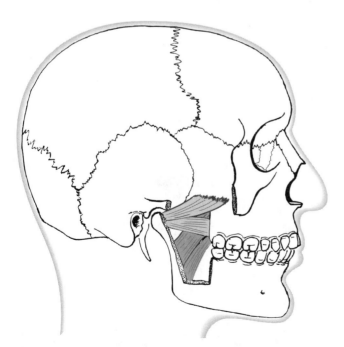

FIGURE 14-8 Label medial and lateral pterygoid muscles.

7. For the temporomandibular joint, give the following information:

Joint	Shape	Degrees of Freedom	Motions
TMJ			

8. At the temporomandibular joint, identify which surface is concave and which is convex.

Joint	Concave	Convex
TMJ		

9. For the temporomandibular joint, provide the close-packed position and the loose-packed position (refer to Chapter 4, Table 4-4).

Joint	Close-Packed	Loose-Packed
TMJ		

10. For the temporomandibular joint, describe the normal end feel (refer to Chapter 4 for descriptions).

For elevation (mouth closing):

_____ Bony   _____ Soft tissue stretch
_____ Soft tissue approximation

For all other motions:

_____ Bony   _____ Soft tissue stretch
_____ Soft tissue approximation

11. Describe the shape and function of the articular disk of the TMJ.

_____

_____

_____

_____

_____

12. Which nerve innervates the muscles that elevate the mandible?

_____

_____

■ ■ ■ Lab Activities

Student's Name _____

Date Due _____

1. Palpation of bones and landmarks, ligaments and other structures:
   • Locate the following structures on bones or skeleton, and palpate on your partner.

TMJ	Located just anterior to the middle anterior part of the ear. Palpate the depression between the mandibular condyle and temporal fossa as your partner opens his or her mouth.

FIGURE 14-9 Palpating the TMJ.

Mandible or Mandibular Bone

Angle	Located between the body and ramus, it is the joining point of these two landmarks. Palpate by placing one finger on the posterior vertical surface of the mandible below the ear and another finger on the posterior horizontal surface. The point (angle) between your fingers is the angle.

FIGURE 14-10 Palpating the angle of the mandible.

Body	The horizontal portion of the mandible. The superior surface of the body holds the teeth. Palpate below the lower teeth on the flat jawline.

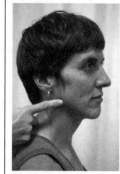

FIGURE 14-11 Palpating the body of the mandible.

Condyle or condylar process	Posterior projection on the ramus that articulates with the temporal bone. Palpate just anterior to the ear canal and inferior to the zygomatic arch while the mouth is open and while the mouth is closed.
Coronoid process	Located anterior to the condyle on the ramus. It is the attachment for the masseter muscle. Palpate below the zygomatic arch while the mouth is fully open. When the mouth is closed, the process moves under the arch and cannot be palpated.
Mental spine	Located on the interior side of the mandible near the midline. It is the attachment for the geniohyoid muscle. Cannot be palpated.
Neck	Located just inferior to the condyle and can be palpated there.
Notch	Located between the condyle and coronoid process on the ramus. Palpate on the ramus of the mandible between the condyle and coronoid process when the mouth is fully open.
Ramus	The vertical portion of the mandible from the angle to the condyle. Palpate on the mandible between the condyle and the angle.

Temporal Bone

Articular tubercle	The anterior portion of the articulating surface of the temporal bone. Difficult to palpate because of overlying muscles.
Articular fossa or mandibular fossa	Located anterior to the external auditory meatus and articulates with the condyle of the mandible. Palpate when the mouth opens; this is not easily palpated.
Postglenoid tubercle	The posterior wall of the fossa just anterior to the external auditory meatus. Not easily palpated because of overlying muscles.
Styloid process	A slender projection positioned down and forward from the temporal bone on the inferior, slightly interior surface. It is the attachment for muscles and ligaments. Palpate behind the earlobe between the mastoid process and ramus of the mandible; it is difficult to palpate because of overlying muscles.
Mastoid process	Large bony prominence posterior and inferior to the ear. It is an attachment for digastric and sternocleidomastoid muscles. Palpate just posterior to the ear.

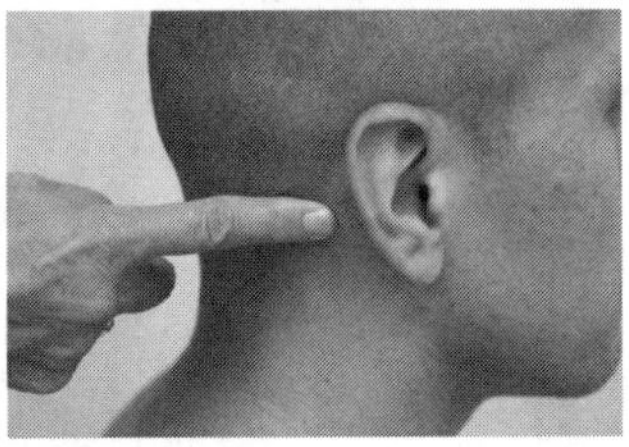

FIGURE 14-12 Palpating the mastoid process.

External auditory meatus	External opening for the ear, located posterior to the TMJ. View from lateral side of head.
Zygomatic process	Posterior portion of the zygomatic arch. It is the attachment for the masseter. Palpate just anterior to the ear on the zygomatic arch.

Sphenoid Bone*

Greater wing	Large bony process located medial to the zygomatic bone and arch and anterior to the rest of the temporal bone. It is the attachment for the temporalis and lateral pterygoid muscles.
Lateral pterygoid plate	Deep to the zygomatic arch. It is the attachment for the lateral and medial pterygoid muscles.
Spine	Deep to the articular fossa of the temporal bone. It is the attachment for the sphenomandibular ligament.

*Because the sphenoid is located inside the cranium, none of the following structures can be palpated.

Combination of Skull Bones

Temporal fossa	Bony floor formed by zygomatic, frontal, parietal, sphenoid, and temporal bones. It is the attachment for the temporalis muscle. Palpate the general area of the fossa above the ear and zygomatic arch.
Zygomatic arch	Formed by the zygomatic process of the temporal bone posteriorly and the temporal process of the zygomatic bone anteriorly. Palpate anterior to the external auditory meatus between the temporalis and zygomatic bones along the arch. 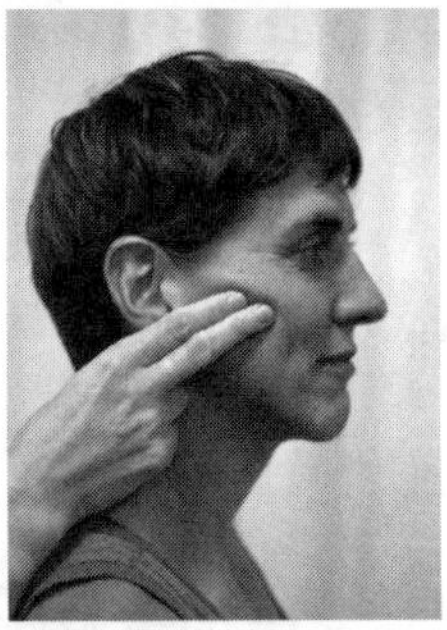

FIGURE 14-13 Palpating the zygomatic arch.

Maxilla or Maxillary Bone

Tuberosity	Rounded projection located on the inferior posterior angle. It is the attachment for the medial pterygoid. Cannot be palpated.

Other Structures

Hyoid bone	Horseshoe-shaped bone lying superior to the thyroid cartilage at about the C3 level. It is the attachment for the stylohyoid ligaments, tongue, suprahyoid, and infrahyoid muscles. Palpate on either side of the trachea parallel to the jaw. Notice how it elevates when your partner swallows.

FIGURE 14-14 Palpating the hyoid bone.

Thyroid cartilage or "Adam's apple"	Inferior to the hyoid bone at about the C3 to C4 level. It is the attachment for the infrahyoid muscles. This structure is more pronounced in males than in females. Palpate in the midline below the hyoid bone.
Lateral ligament or temporomandibular ligament	Attaches on the neck of the mandibular condyle and disk, and then runs superiorly to the articular tubercle of the temporal bone. Cannot be palpated.
Sphenomandibular ligament	Attaches to the spine of the sphenoid bone and runs to the middle of the ramus on the internal surface of the mandible. Cannot be palpated.

Stylomandibular ligament	Attaches to the styloid process of the temporal bone and to the posterior inferior border of the ramus of the mandible. Cannot be palpated.
Stylohyoid ligament	Attaches to the styloid process of the temporal bone and the hyoid bone. Deep to muscles and cannot be palpated.
Joint capsule	Envelops the TMJ. Attaches superiorly to the articular tubercle and borders of the temporal bone, and attaches inferiorly to the neck of the condyle of the mandible. Cannot be palpated.
Articular disk	Attached circumferentially to the capsule and tendon of the lateral pterygoid. Palpate by placing a finger in the external auditory meatus while your partner opens/closes his or her mouth.

2. Palpation of muscles:

   A. Locate the following muscles on the skeleton, anatomical models, and on at least one partner.

      • The information needed to palpate each muscle is provided in the following tables.

      • The position described for locating the muscle on your partner is usually the manual muscle test position for a fair or better grade of muscle strength.

      • Not all origins, insertions, and muscle bellies can be palpated on your partner.

   B. On the skeleton, locate the origin and insertion of each muscle.

      • Place the ends of a rubber band at the origin and insertion of the muscle, making the band taut. Note the location of the muscle in relation to the joints it crosses.

Sitting Position

TEMPORALIS:	Superficial on the lateral aspect of the skull

FIGURE 14-15 Palpating the temporalis.

Position of person:	Mouth open
Origin:	Temporal fossa
Insertion:	Coronoid process and ramus of mandible
Line of pull:	Anterior fibers—vertical; middle fibers—diagonal; posterior fibers—horizontal
Muscle action:	Bilaterally: Elevation and retrusion Unilaterally: Ipsilateral lateral deviation
Palpate:	On the lateral aspect of the skull above the TMJ
Instructions to person:	While palpating bilaterally, say, "Close your mouth." While palpating on the left, say, "Move your jaw to the left."
MASSETER:	One part is superficial and the other is deep; located in the posterior portion of the cheek between the mandibular angle and zygomatic arch

FIGURE 14-16 Palpating the masseter.

Position of person:	Mouth closed but jaw relaxed
Origin:	Zygomatic arch of temporal bone and zygomatic process of maxilla
Insertion:	Angle of ramus and coronoid process of mandible
Line of pull:	Mostly vertical
Muscle action:	Bilaterally: Elevation Unilaterally: Ipsilateral lateral deviation
Palpate:	Over the posterior part of the cheek below the zygomatic arch
Instructions to person:	While palpating bilaterally or unilaterally, say, "Clench and relax your jaw."
MEDIAL PTERYGOID:	On the inside of the mandibular ramus
Position of person:	Mouth open
Origin:	Lateral pterygoid plate of the sphenoid bone and tuberosity of the maxilla
Insertion:	Ramus and angle of the mandible
Line of pull:	Diagonal
Muscle action:	Bilaterally: Elevation, protrusion Unilaterally: Contralateral lateral deviation
Palpate:	Difficult but may possibly be palpated from inside the mouth. Wearing examination gloves, place your index finger inside the mouth and your thumb outside on the mandible. To distinguish from the masseter, have the person laterally deviate to the opposite side.
Instructions to person:	While palpating the right medial pterygoid, say, "Move your jaw to the left."
LATERAL PTERYGOID:	Deep
Position of person:	Mouth closed
Origin:	Lateral pterygoid plate and greater wing of the sphenoid
Insertion:	Mandibular condyle and articular disk
Line of pull:	Horizontal
Muscle action:	Bilaterally: Depression, protrusion Unilaterally: Contralateral lateral deviation

Palpate:	Difficult but may possibly be palpated from inside the mouth. Wearing examination gloves, place your index finger inside the mouth behind the molars on the maxilla and your thumb outside in the same place. To distinguish from the masseter, have the person laterally deviate to the opposite side.
Instructions to person:	While palpating the right lateral pterygoid, say, "Open your mouth and move your jaw to the left."
SUPRAHYOIDS:	Form a wall of muscles along the underside of the jaw between the mandible and the hyoid bone. All insert on the hyoid bone.
Mylohyoid	Deep. Origin: Interior medial mandible
Geniohyoid	Deep. Origin: Mental spine of mandible
Stylohyoid	Deep: Origin: Styloid process of temporal bone
Insertion:	All on the hyoid bone
Muscle action:	Assists in depressing mandible
Palpate:	Place your fingers along the underside of the mandible. Distinguishing between the individual suprahyoid muscles is difficult.
Instructions to person:	While palpating the suprahyoid group, say, "Press the tip of your tongue against the roof of your mouth."
Digastric	Deep
Position of person:	Mouth closed
Origin:	Anterior: Internal inferior mandible Posterior: Mastoid process
Insertion:	Hyoid
Muscle action:	Assists in depressing mandible

Palpate:	Place one finger on the mastoid process and another finger on the hyoid bone. Draw an imaginary line between the two points and place your fingers along this line. Place another finger under the person's chin.
Instructions to person:	While palpating the digastric, say, "Open your mouth against my finger."
INFRAHYOIDS:	Located below the hyoid bone. For the TMJ, they serve to stabilize the hyoid so that the suprahyoid muscles can depress the mandible. All but the sternothyroid insert on the inferior border of the hyoid bone. The sternothyroid inserts on the thyroid cartilage.
Sternohyoid	Deep. Origin: Medial end of clavicle, sternoclavicular ligament, manubrium of sternum
Sternothyroid	Deep. Origin: Manubrium of sternum and cartilage of the first rib
Thyrohyoid	Deep. Origin: Thyroid cartilage
Omohyoid	Deep. Origin: Superior border of the scapula
Muscle action:	Stabilizes the hyoid bone
Palpate:	Difficult to distinguish between the sternohyoid and sternothyroid. Place your fingers alongside the trachea, just below the thyroid cartilage (Adam's apple) and medial to the sternocleidomastoid muscle. Use your other hand over the forehead to resist head and neck flexion.
Instructions to person:	Bring your chin to your chest.

3. Perform the motions of the temporomandibular joint on yourself and on your partner.

   A. Place your index fingers just anterior to your auditory canals. You can feel the movement of the TMJ as you open and close your mouth, move it from side to side, and move it forward and back.

   B. Perform a motion and then your partner names the motion you performed.

   C. Your partner states a motion and then you perform that motion.

4. Observe the amount of motion in each direction at the temporomandibular joint. Motion of the TMJ is often measured with a ruler and recorded in inches or millimeters. For each of the motions available at the TMJ joint, estimate the amount of motion available.

Motions	Inches/Millimeters
Protrusion	
Depression (opening)	
Lateral deviation to one side	

5. Individuals often have difficulty allowing passive movement of the mandible. Passively move your partner through the available range of motion, making note of the end feel. If possible, repeat with several people. Review question 10 in the pre-lab worksheets about normal end feels for the motions of the TMJ.

   A. Is your partner's end feel consistent with normal end feel? _____

   B. What structures create the end feel for this joint? _____

6. Use a disarticulated skeleton or an anatomical model of the temporomandibular joint and apply the rules of joint arthrokinematics and the concave-convex rule to perform the following activities:

   A. Underline the correct answer.
   The temporal bone is concave/convex.
   The mandible condyle is concave/convex.

   B. Move the mandible on the temporal bone in all planes of motion.

   C. Observe the movement of the mandible on the temporal bone. Circle the motions that you observe.

   Roll   Spin   Glide

7. People without proper head alignment may have difficulty swallowing and often choke when eating. Also, they may drool. Use caution performing the following activities. Make note of the ease of drinking and eating in each position. In the following three positions, take a drink of water and eat a cracker or cookie.

   • Position 1: With head, neck, and trunk in proper alignment

   • Position 2: With head, neck, and trunk in flexion

   • Position 3: With head, neck, and trunk in full extension

   A. In which position(s) was it easy to drink and eat? _____

   B. In which position(s) was it difficult to drink and eat? _____

   C. Explain. _____

   _____

8. Which motions of the TMJ do people typically use when chewing?

   _____

9. Biting off a piece of jerky requires which TMJ muscles to perform what type of contraction(s)?

   _____

10. An acrobat is hanging and spinning, supported only by biting on a mouthpiece.

   A. Which TMJ motion(s) would definitely not be wanted? _____

   B. Which TMJ muscle(s) would prevent this unwanted motion? _____

■ ■ ■ Post-Lab Questions

Student's Name _____

Date Due _____

After you have completed the worksheets and lab activities, answer the following questions without using your book or notes. When finished, check your answers.

1. For each muscle listed, check the motions for which the muscle is considered a prime mover.

Muscle	Elevation	Depression	Protrusion	Retrusion	Ipsilateral Lateral Deviation	Contralateral Lateral Deviation
Temporalis						
Masseter						
Medial pterygoid						
Lateral pterygoid						

2. What motions of the TMJ will be absent if cranial nerve V is severed?

_____

3. Describe the movement of the articular disk during left lateral deviation of the mandible.

_____

4. Bell's palsy is a condition resulting from insult to facial nerve, or cranial nerve, VII. The injury to the nerve is thought to occur as it exits a foramen in the mandible. Which TMJ muscles will be affected by an injury to cranial nerve VII? _____

5. What muscle lies deep to the masseter muscle? _____

6. The TMJ is which type of joint? Describe. _____

7. Which cranial nerve provides motor innervation to muscles of mastication? _____

8. Which cranial nerve provides motor innervation to the sternocleidomastoid and trapezius?

_____

9. Which cranial nerve provides motor innervation to muscles of facial expression?

_____

10. On Figure 14-17, identify the areas of the head and face innervated by cranial nerve V:

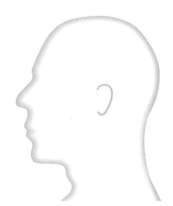

FIGURE 14-17 Innervated area of trigeminal nerve.

11. Describe what occurs in the two phases of mandibular depression (opening the jaw).

_____

_____

Neck and Trunk

■ ■ ■ Pre-Lab Worksheets

Student's Name _____

Date Due _____

Complete the following questions prior to the lab class.

1. Define the following terms:

   Spine: _____

   Facet: _____

2. A. An increase in the curvature of the thoracic spine in the sagittal plane is referred to as _____.

   B. Increased curvature of the lumbar spine in the sagittal plane is referred to as _____.

3. Indicate on Figure 15-1 the cervical, thoracic, lumbar, and sacral regions of the spine. Which of these regions are concave and which are convex anteriorly?

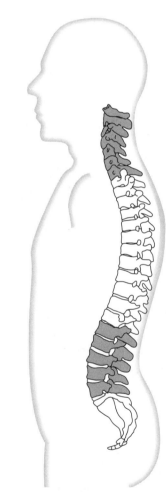

FIGURE 15-1 Vertebral column.

4. On Figures 15-2 through 15-7, label the following bones and landmarks:

BONES: Occipital Mandible Maxilla Parietal

Frontal Temporal Sphenoid Zygomatic

LANDMARKS: Basilar Foramen Mastoid

area magnum process

Occipital External auditory

condyle meatus

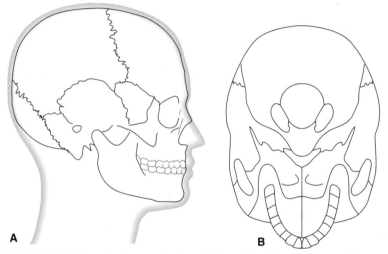

FIGURE 15-2 The skull, lateral view, **(A)** and skull base, viewed from below **(B)**.

LANDMARKS ON VERTEBRA:

Body Neural arch Vertebral
foramen

Articular process Pedicle Lamina

Transverse process Spinous process

VERTEBRAL Intervertebral Intervertebral Facet
JOINT: foramen disk joint

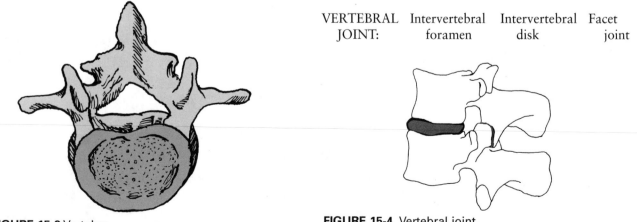

FIGURE 15-3 Vertebra.

FIGURE 15-4 Vertebral joint.

ATLAS: Anterior   Posterior   Articular   THORACIC   Facet   Demifacet   Vertebral
         arch   arch   process   VERTEBRAE: (three   body
                                                                       shown)
         Transverse   Vertebral   Transverse   Spinous   Rib
         process   foramen   foramen   process

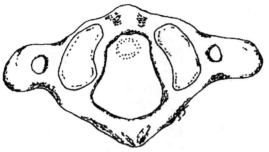

FIGURE 15-5 Superior view of the atlas.

AXIS: Dens   Transverse   Superior   Body
                   foramen   articular
                                  process

        Lamina   Spinous   Transverse
                   process   process

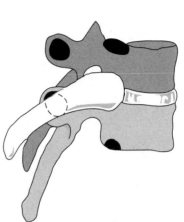

FIGURE 15-7 Thoracic vertebrae.

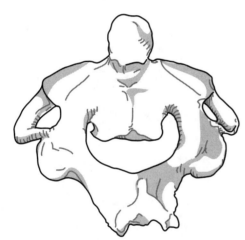

FIGURE 15-6 Posterior view of the axis.

5. On Figure 15-8, label the following structures:

Body	Spinous process
Anterior longitudinal ligament	Posterior longitudinal ligament
Supraspinal ligament	Interspinal ligament
Ligamentum flavum	Lamina

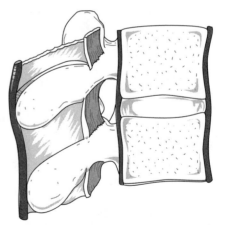

FIGURE 15-8 Vertebral parts and ligaments.

6. On Figure 15-9, label the three parts of the scalene muscle.

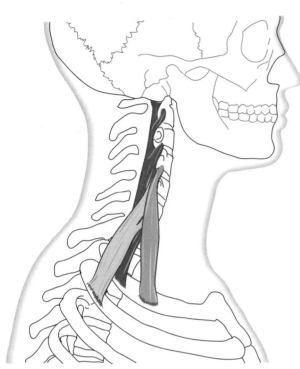

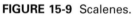

FIGURE 15-9 Scalenes.

7. On Figures 15-10 through 15-14:

A. Label the origin and insertion of the muscles listed.

B. Join the origin and insertion to show the line of pull.

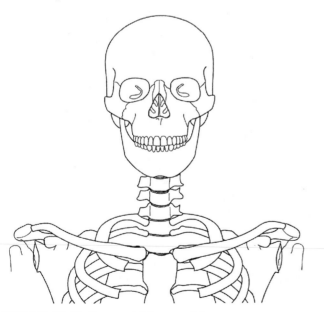

FIGURE 15-10 Sternocleidomastoid.

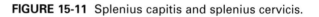

FIGURE 15-11 Splenius capitis and splenius cervicis.

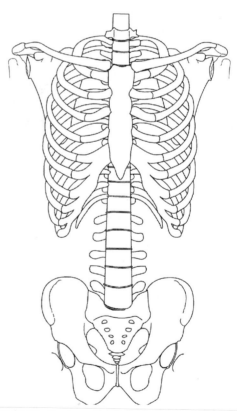

FIGURE 15-12 Rectus abdominis and I transverse abdominis.

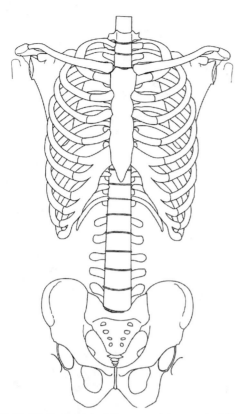

FIGURE 15-13 External oblique and internal oblique.

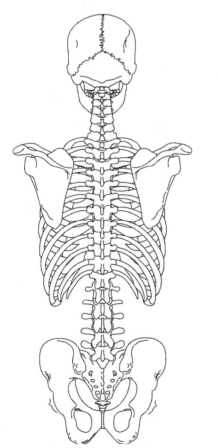

FIGURE 15-14 Quadratus lumborum and erector spinae.

8. For each of the joints listed, give the following information:

Joint	Degrees of Freedom	Motions	Plane	Axis
Atlanto-occipital				
Atlantoaxial				

9. For the following joints, identify which surface is concave and which is convex.

Joint	Concave	Convex
Atlanto-occipital		
Atlantoaxial		

10. Facet joints are formed by the articulation between the _____ articular processes of the vertebra below with the _____ articular processes of the vertebra above.

11. What determines the extent, the type, and the amount of motion possible at each part of the vertebral column? _____

12. What limits spinal motion in the thoracic region?

    _____

13. Trunk lateral bending occurs in the _____ plane about the _____ axis.

■ ■ ■ Lab Activities

Student's Name _____

Date Due _____

1. Palpation of bones and landmarks, ligaments, and other structures:
   - Locate the following structures on bones or skeleton, and palpate on your partner when possible.
   - Most of these structures cannot be palpated.
   - The reference position is the anatomical position.

Skull

Occipital bone or occiput	Posterior inferior part of the skull. The area above the occipital protuberance is superficial. The part below curves in under the head and is covered by muscles. Putting your hand on the back of your head covers much of the occiput.
Occipital protuberance	The small prominence in the center of the occiput. Palpate over the skull in the midline of the occiput.

FIGURE 15-15 Palpating the occipital protuberance.

Basilar area	Base, or inferior, portion of the occiput. Cannot be palpated.
Foramen magnum	Opening in the occipital bone through which the spinal cord enters the cranium. Cannot be palpated.

Occipital condyles	Located laterally to the foramen magnum on the occiput; articulates with atlas. Cannot be palpated.
Temporal bone	Forms part of the base and lateral inferior sides of the cranium. Palpate on the side of the head just anterior and superior to the ear.
Mastoid process	Bony prominence behind the earlobe; attachment for the sternocleidomastoid. Palpate just behind the ear (see Fig. 14-12).

Vertebra

Body	Anterior portion of the vertebra; C1 and C2 do not have a body. Cannot be palpated.
Neural arch or vertebral arch	Posterior portion of the vertebra. Cannot be palpated. Only the transverse and spinous processes can be palpated.
Vertebral foramen	Opening formed by the joining of the body and neural arch through which the spinal cord passes. Cannot be palpated.
Pedicle	Portion of the neural arch posterior to the body and anterior to the lamina. Cannot be palpated.
Lamina	Posterior portion of the neural arch that unites from each side of the midline. Cannot be palpated.

Continued

Vertebra—Cont'd

Transverse process	Formed at the union of the lamina and pedicle, the lateral projections of the arch to which muscles and ligaments attach. Palpate on the lateral aspect of the neck inferior to the earlobes.

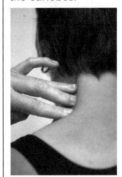

FIGURE 15-16 Cervical transverse processes.

Vertebral notches	Depressions located on the superior and inferior surfaces of the pedicle. Cannot be palpated.
Intervertebral foramen	Opening formed by the superior notch of the vertebra below and the inferior notch of the vertebra above. Cannot be palpated.
Articular process	Projecting superiorly and inferiorly off the posterior surface of each lamina. Superior articular processes face posteriorly or medially whereas the inferior processes face anteriorly or laterally. Cannot be palpated.
Spinous process	Most posterior projection on the neural arch; located at the junction of the two laminae. It is the attachment for many muscles and ligaments. The tips of spinous processes can be palpated as a ridge in the midline of the back. In the cervical area, the spinous processes can be palpated under the ligamentum nuchae when the neck is in hyperextension. The spinous processes can also be palpated in the thoracic and lumbar regions.

Intervertebral Disk

Annulus fibrosus	The outer portion of the disk consisting of several concentrically arranged fibrocartilaginous rings. Cannot be palpated.
Nucleus pulposus	Pulpy gelatinous substance with high water content in the center of the disk. Cannot be palpated.

Atlas

Atlas C1	The first cervical vertebra upon which the cranium rests. Round without a body or a spinous process. Cannot be palpated on most people.
Anterior arch	The anterior portion of the atlas. Cannot be palpated.

Axis

Axis C2	Second cervical vertebra. The transverse and spinous processes can be palpated on the side and posterior midline, respectively.
Dens or odontoid process	Large vertical projection located anteriorly on the axis. Cannot be palpated.

Other Structures

C7 or vertebra prominens	Has a long and prominent spinous process. Easily palpated, and often quite visible with neck flexion.

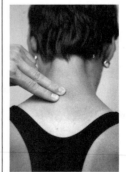

FIGURE 15-17 Palpating C7.

Transverse foramen	Holes in the transverse process of the cervical vertebra through which the vertebral artery passes. Cannot be palpated.
Facet or costal facets	Located superiorly and inferiorly on the sides of the bodies and on transverse processes of thoracic vertebrae. Articulation with ribs. Cannot be palpated.
Demifacet	Partial or half facet; located laterally on the superior and inferior edges of the vertebral body where ribs articulate with thoracic vertebrae. Cannot be palpated.

2. Palpation of joints and ligaments:

Atlanto-occipital joint	Joint of first cervical vertebra and occiput. Cannot be palpated.
Atlantoaxial joints	Joint between C1 and C2. Cannot be palpated.
Median atlantoaxial joints	Synovial articulation between the dens (odontoid) process of the axis and the anterior arch of the atlas anteriorly and the transverse ligament posteriorly. Cannot be palpated.
Lateral atlantoaxial joints	Joints between the articular processes of two vertebrae. Cannot be palpated.
Facet joints	Articulations on posterior and lateral aspects of the vertebrae; the superior articular process of the vertebra below and the inferior articular process of the vertebra above. Cannot be palpated.
Anterior longitudinal ligament	Located on the anterior surface of the bodies of the vertebral column. Cannot be palpated.

Posterior longitudinal ligament	Located on the posterior surface of the vertebral bodies in the vertebral foramen. Cannot be palpated.
Supraspinal ligament	Located posteriorly along the tips of the spinous processes extending from C7 to sacrum. Palpate by placing fingertips between two adjacent thoracic or lumbar spinous processes and having the person slightly flex the trunk. This movement causes the ligament to become taut.
Ligamentum nuchae or nuchal ligament	Located posteriorly along the tips of the spinous processes in the cervical region. Palpate by placing fingertips between two adjacent cervical spinous processes and having the person slightly flex the neck. This movement causes the ligament to become taut.

FIGURE 15-18 Palpating the nuchal ligament.

Interspinal ligament	Joins the spinous processes of adjacent vertebrae by attaching to the under surface of the spinous process above and the upper surface of the spinous process below. Cannot be palpated.
Ligamentum flavum	Located on the anterior surface of the neural arch inside the vertebral foramen. Cannot be palpated.

3. Palpation of muscles

   A. Locate the following muscles on at least one partner, the skeleton, and anatomical models.

   - The information needed to palpate each muscle is provided in the following tables.
   - The position described for locating the muscle on your partner is usually the manual muscle test position for a fair or better grade of muscle strength.
   - Not all origins, insertions, and muscle bellies can be palpated.

   B. On the skeleton, locate the origin and insertion of each muscle.

   - Place the ends of a rubber band at the origin and insertion of the muscle, making the rubber band taut. Note the location of the muscle in relation to the joints it crosses.
   - When possible, move the skeleton to perform the muscle's motion and observe how the band becomes less taut, similar to the change in length as it performs a concentric contraction.

Supine Position

STERNOCLEIDOMASTOID:	Located superficially on anterior aspect of neck
	FIGURE 15-19 Palpating the right sternocleidomastoid muscle. FIGURE 15-20 Both sternocleidomastoid muscles.
Position of person:	Unilateral: Head turned to one side Bilateral: Head in midline

Origin:	Sternum and clavicle
Insertion:	Mastoid process
Line of pull:	Diagonal
Muscle action:	Unilaterally: Laterally bends neck; rotates head to opposite side Bilaterally: Flexes neck, and hyperextends head
Palpate:	Anterior aspect of neck between the sternal end of the clavicle and the mastoid process
Instructions to person:	Unilaterally, say, "Looking to the side, lift your head off the table." Bilaterally, say, "Looking ahead, lift your head off the table."
SCALENES:	Deep on lateral aspect of neck FIGURE 15-21 Palpating the right scalene muscles.
Position of person:	Head in the midline
Origin:	Anterior scalene: Transverse processes of C3–C6 Middle scalene: Transverse processes of C2–C7 Posterior scalene: Transverse processes of C5–C7
Insertion:	Anterior scalene: Superior surface of the first rib Middle scalene: Superior surface of the first rib Posterior scalene: Second rib
Line of pull:	Vertical
Muscle action:	Unilaterally: Laterally bend neck Bilaterally: Assists with neck flexion

Palpate:	On lateral aspect of neck between the sternocleidomastoid and the upper trapezius, giving slight resistance to lateral bending
Instructions to person:	Unilaterally, say, "Move your ear toward your shoulder." Bilaterally, say, "Lift your head off the table."
RECTUS ABDOMINIS:	Located superficially on abdomen

FIGURE 15-22 Palpating the rectus abdominis muscle.

Position of person:	Arms at sides
Origin:	Pubis
Insertion:	Costal cartilages of fifth, sixth, and seventh ribs
Line of pull:	Vertical on the anterior trunk
Muscle action:	Trunk flexion
Palpate:	Midline of abdomen
Instructions to person:	Curl your body until your scapulae are off the table.
EXTERNAL OBLIQUE:	Located superficially on lateral aspect of abdomen

FIGURE 15-23 Palpating the right external oblique muscle.

Position of person:	Arms at sides
Origin:	Lower eight ribs laterally
Insertion:	Iliac crest and linea alba

Line of pull:	Diagonal on the anterior trunk
Muscle action:	Unilaterally: Lateral bending; rotation to opposite side Bilaterally: Trunk flexion; compression of abdomen
Palpate:	On the right lateral abdomen for right external oblique muscle
Instructions to person:	Reach toward your left hip, rotating your right shoulder off the table. (Subject in photo is not reaching so that the arm does not obstruct the view of where to palpate.)
INTERNAL OBLIQUE:	Located deep to external oblique muscle

FIGURE 15-24 Palpating the left internal oblique.

Position of person:	Arms at sides
Origin:	Inguinal ligament, iliac crest, thoracolumbar fascia
Insertion:	Tenth, 11th, and 12th ribs, abdominal aponeurosis
Line of pull:	Diagonal on the anterior trunk.
Muscle action:	Unilaterally: Lateral bending; rotation to same side Bilaterally: Trunk flexion; compression of the abdomen
Palpate:	On left lateral abdomen for left internal oblique muscle, deep to the left external oblique
Instructions to person:	Reach toward your left hip while rotating your right shoulder off the table. Left external oblique is not contracting during this motion. (Subject in photo is not reaching so that the arm does not obstruct the view of where to palpate.)

Continued

Supine Position—Cont'd

TRANSVERSE ABDOMINIS:	Deep to the oblique muscles
Position of person:	Arms at sides
Origin:	Inguinal ligament, iliac crest, thoracolumbar fascia, and last six ribs
Insertion:	Abdominal aponeurosis and linea alba
Line of pull:	Horizontal on the anterior trunk
Muscle action:	Compression of abdomen
Palpate:	Lateral aspect of abdomen. Cannot be differentiated from other more superficial anterior trunk muscles.
Instructions to person:	Cough.
PREVERTEBRAL:	Deep on anterior aspect of neck
Position of person:	Head in midline
Origin:	Collectively, from bodies and transverse processes of upper cervical vertebra
Insertion:	Collectively, to occipital bone and transverse processes and bodies of upper cervical vertebra
Line of pull:	Vertical on the anterior trunk
Muscle action:	Flex head on C1
Palpate:	Cannot be palpated
Instruction to person:	Tuck your chin.
QUADRATUS LUMBORUM:	Deep
Position of person:	Good postural alignment
Origin:	Iliac crest
Insertion:	12th rib, transverse processes of all five lumbar vertebrae
Line of pull:	Vertical on the lateral side of the trunk
Muscle action:	Trunk lateral bending; hip hiking (elevation of one side of the pelvis)
Palpate:	Difficult to palpate. May be possible on a thin person by palpating very deep on the lateral side of the torso between the lower ribs and the iliac crest.
Instructions to person:	Slide the left side of your pelvis toward your left shoulder, keeping your pelvis on the table.

Prone Position

SPLENIUS CAPITIS/ CERVICIS:	Deep to trapezius and levator scapula
Position of person:	Head in midline, shoulders parallel to the pelvis
Origin:	Capitis: Lower half of nuchal ligament; spinous processes of C7 through T3 Cervicis: Spinous processes of T3 through T6
Insertion:	Capitis: Lateral occipital bone; mastoid process Cervicis: Transverse processes of C1 through C3
Line of pull:	Capitis: Diagonal Cervicis: Vertical
Muscle action:	Capitis: Unilaterally: Laterally bend and rotate head to same side Bilaterally: Extend neck Cervicis: Unilaterally: Laterally bend and rotate face to same side Bilaterally: Extend neck
Palpate:	Difficult to palpate, as they are deep to the erector spinae
Instructions to person:	Unilaterally, say, "Tilt your head and turn your head to the right." Bilaterally, say, "Lift your head up and look straight ahead."

ERECTOR SPINAE:	Located along the vertebral column from neck to lumbar region. Some are deep and some are superficial.

FIGURE 15-25 Palpating the erector spinae muscle.

Position of person:	Head in midline, shoulders parallel to the pelvis
Origin:	Spinalis group: Nuchal ligament and spinous processes of cervical and thoracic vertebrae Longissimus group: Transverse processes from occiput to sacrum Iliocostalis group: Sacrum, ilium, and ribs
Insertion:	Spinalis group: Occiput and transverse processes Longissimus group: Transverse processes and adjacent ribs Iliocostalis group: Transverse processes to C7 and the ribs
Line of pull:	Vertical
Muscle action:	Unilaterally: Lateral bending of neck and trunk Bilaterally: Extend neck and trunk
Palpate:	Posterior neck and trunk: Spinalis group is medial, iliocostalis group is lateral, and longissimus group is between the other two. Difficult to differentiate.
Instructions to person:	Unilaterally, say, "Move your ear toward your shoulder." Bilaterally, say, "Lift your head off the table."
TRANSVERSOSPINALIS:	Posterior, deep to erector spinae. Three muscles: Semispinalis, multifidus, rotators.

Position of person:	Head in midline, shoulders parallel to the pelvis
Origin:	Transverse processes
Insertion:	Spinous processes of vertebra above
Line of pull:	Diagonal on the posterior side of the trunk
Muscle action:	Unilaterally: Rotation to opposite side Bilaterally: Extend trunk
Palpate:	Cannot be palpated
Instruction to observe muscle action:	Unilaterally: To examine left muscles, say, "Raise your head and right shoulder off the table." Bilaterally, say, "Look up and lift your head and trunk off the table."
INTERSPINALES AND INTERTRANSVERSARII:	Posterior, deep to erector spinae
Position of person:	Head in midline, shoulders parallel to the pelvis
Origin:	Interspinales: Spinous process below Intertransversarii: Transverse process below
Insertion:	Interspinales: Spinous process above Intertransversarii: Transverse process above
Line of pull:	Vertical on the posterior side of the trunk
Muscle action:	Intertransversarii: Neck and trunk lateral bending Interspinales: Neck and trunk extension
Palpate:	Cannot be palpated
Instruction to observe muscle action:	Unilaterally: To examine left muscles, say, "Slide your left shoulder toward your left pelvis, keeping your trunk on the table." Bilaterally, say, "Look up and lift your head and trunk off the table."

4. Perform the motions of the neck and trunk with your partner.

   A. Perform a motion and then your partner names the motion you performed.

   B. Your partner states a motion and you perform that motion.

5. Observe your partner flex, extend, laterally bend, and rotate. Indicate the amount of motion available in each of the three regions of the spinal column as minimal or maximum.

Spinal Region	Flexion/ Extension	Lateral Bending	Rotation
Cervical			
Thoracic			
Lumbar			

6. Perform the following two variations of sit-ups. Determine if the position of the hips makes a difference in performing the sit-up and explain your answer. Sit up only until scapula clears the table. Start with the arms at the side reaching forward as the sit-up is performed.

   A. With hips and knees flexed so feet are close to buttocks

   B. With legs extended

   _____

   _____

   _____

   _____

7. Perform the following variations of a sit-up to determine which is the easiest and which is the hardest. Explain why.

   A. Hands overhead

   B. Hands crossed over chest

   C. Arms extended in front

   _____

   _____

8. Perform trunk flexion (trunk curl) in supine position. Compare the range of trunk motion achieved with the range of motion achieved in questions 7 and 8.

   A. Where does the additional ROM come from in the sit-up exercises in question 7?

   _____

   B. Which method, sit up or trunk curl, is less likely to increase lumbar lordosis? Explain your answer.

   _____ Sit-up _____ Trunk curl

9. With your partner lying on a table with hands on shoulders and legs extended, place one of your hands under your partner's lower lumbar region. Place your other hand on your partner's abdomen. Ask your partner to press the low back into the table. Complete the following:

   A.

Motion Performed	Agonist	Antagonist
Trunk flexion		

   B. If your partner is unable to press the low back into the table, which muscles may be too short to permit the movement to occur? _____

   C. If your partner is unable to press the low back into the table, which muscles may be too weak or long to perform the movement? _____

10. In the standing position, slide your left hand down the side of your leg, thereby bringing your shoulder closer to your knee.

    A. What motion did you perform? _____

    B. Which muscle(s) performed the motion? _____

    C. What type of contraction has the agonist performed?

    _____ Eccentric _____ Concentric

11. Apply paper tape strips to your partner's abdomen to represent the layers of the abdominal muscles. Apply the strips from the origin to the insertion of each muscle. Write the name of the muscle on each tape. Ensure that the tape strip "muscles" are applied in the correct layer.

12. In each of the activities, identify which muscles are the agonists. Starting in the supine position:

   A. With the head in midline, ask your partner to flex the head and neck only. _____

   B. With the head in midline, ask your partner to tuck the chin. _____

   C. With the head turned to the left, ask you partner to lift the head off the table.

   _____

13. With your partner sitting and facing you, palpate the carotid artery in the space between the thyroid cartilage (Adam's Apple) and the SCM muscle. Because this artery supplies much of the blood to the brain, be cautious: Do not palpate both sides at the same time!

■ ■ ■ Post-Lab Questions

Student's Name _____

Date Due _____

After you have completed the worksheets and lab activities, answer the following questions without using your book or notes. When finished, check your answers.

1. List the other terms also used to describe the following bones or landmarks:

   A. Dens: _____

   B. Seventh cervical vertebra: _____

   C. First cervical vertebra: _____

   D. Second cervical vertebra: _____

   E. Neural arch: _____

2. Which vertebra does not have a spinous process or a body? _____

3. C1 articulates with which landmark of the skull?

   _____

4. What position does the head assume when the left sternocleidomastoid performs a concentric contraction?

   ____ Lateral bending with rotation to the right
   ____ Lateral bending with rotation to the left

5. Which pair of oblique muscles performs a sit-up with rotation to the right?

   ____ Right internal and left external oblique
   ____ Left internal and right external oblique

6. When performing bilateral leg raises, which muscle group must perform what type of contraction to prevent the low back from arching?

   _____

   _____

7. What muscle groups make up the erector spinae muscle group?

   _____

   _____

8. The quadratus lumborum performs a _____ contraction during hip hiking and an _____ contraction during lateral bending to the _____ side.

9. List the muscles of the posterior cervical region from deepest to most superficial—this includes muscles covered in previous chapters.

   _____

   _____

   _____

   _____

10. Which head/neck muscle is innervated by a cranial nerve and which cranial nerve is it?

    Muscle: _____

    Nerve: _____

11. The suboccipital muscles perform what motions of the head?

    _____

12. When lying supine, a person lifts the head, bringing the chin to the chest.

    A. The motion occurring at the neck is _____.

    B. What is the effect of gravity on the motion?

    _____

    C. The muscles contracting are the neck _____.

    D. The type of contraction is _____.

    E. The axis of motion is _____, while the plane of motion is _____.

13. On Figure 15-26, outline the dermatomes of T2, T7, and T12.

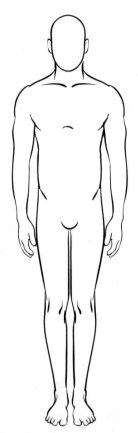

FIGURE 15-26 Anterior view.

Chapter 16

Respiratory System

■ ■ ■ Pre-Lab Worksheets

Student's Name _____

Date Due _____

Complete the following questions prior to the lab class.

1. Match the following phases of respiration with the appropriate definition.

   _____ Quiet inspiration   A. Muscles compress the abdomen

   _____ Deep inspiration   B. Mostly a passive action

   _____ Forced inspiration   C. Uses muscles that pull ribs up

   _____ Quiet expiration   D. Diaphragm and external intercostals are prime movers

   _____ Forced expiration   E. In a state of "air hunger"

2. Describe the differences between diaphragmatic breathing and chest breathing in terms of energy required and amount of air exchanged.

3. A. What is a Valsalva maneuver?

   B. When do people tend to use the Valsalva maneuver?

   C. Describe the series of events that have the potential to cause cardiac disturbance when a person performs a Valsalva maneuver.

4. List the anatomical structures that are referred to as the "bronchial tree."

5. On Figure 16-1, label the following joints, bones, and landmarks:

True ribs   False ribs   Floating ribs   Costal cartilage

Manubrium   Xiphoid process   Sternal body

6. Label the listed structures on the figures.

A. Label the joints and bones on Figure 16-2:

Costovertebral joints   Vertebral body   Rib   Transverse process

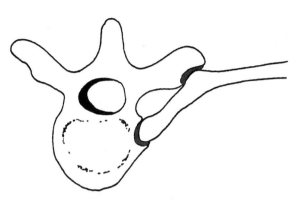

FIGURE 16-2 Costovertebral joint.

B. Identify the following respiratory structures on Figure 16-3:

Larynx   Trachea   Bronchioles
Alveoli   Nasal cavity   Oral cavity
Nasopharynx   Oral pharynx   Diaphragm
Laryngopharynx Mediastinum   Bronchi

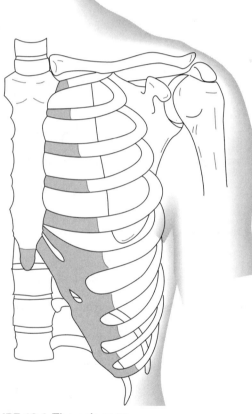

FIGURE 16-1 Thoracic cage.

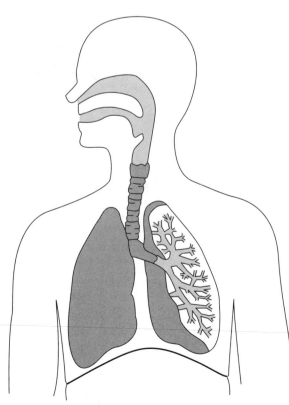

FIGURE 16-3 Respiratory structures.

7. On Figure 16-4:

   A. Label the origin and insertion of the muscles listed.

   B. Join the origin and insertion to show the line of pull.

Diaphragm   External intercostal   Internal intercostal

FIGURE 16-4 Rib cage.

8. At the following joint, identify which surface is concave and which is convex.

Joint	Concave	Convex
Costovertebral		

9. Check the column that indicates the movement of the ribs associated with each phase of respiration.

Phase of Respiration	Elevation	Depression
Inspiration		
Expiration		

10. Describe the function of the soft palate.

   _____

   _____

11. List the three parts of the pharynx.

   _____

   _____

   _____

12. During inspiration, air flows _____ the lungs because the rib cage _____.

   During expiration, air flows _____ the lungs because the rib cage _____.

13. List the accessory muscles of respiration:

Inspiration	Expiration

■ ■ ■ Lab Activities

Student's Name _____

Date Due _____

1. On bones and skeletons, locate, and when possible, palpate on your partner:

   • The reference position is the anatomical position.

   • Not all structures can be palpated on your partner.

Rib Cage	All of the Ribs and Sternum
True ribs	The upper seven ribs. Although difficult, the first rib can be palpated posterior to the clavicle through the scalene muscles. The remaining six ribs can be palpated below the clavicle.
False ribs	Ribs 8–10 attach indirectly to sternum via costal cartilage of the seventh rib. Palpate on the anterior and lateral chest wall.
Floating ribs	Ribs 11–12 have no anterior attachment. Palpate the lateral ends on a person in the prone position. Reach across the person's body to the opposite chest wall. Move your hand inferiorly to the bottom of the rib cage and press deep into soft tissue. The floating ribs are deep to the erector spinae muscles.
Sternum	Palpate in the midline of the anterior chest wall. See Figure 9-12.
Sternal notch	Superior border of sternum between the sternal ends of the clavicles. Palpate between the clavicles at the proximal end of the sternum. See Figure 9-16.
Manubrium	Superior portion of the sternum. As a landmark, it articulates with the clavicle and the first two ribs. Palpate between the sternal notch and body of the sternum. See Figure 9-13.
Body of sternum	Middle portion of the sternum. Palpate between the manubrium and xiphoid process. See Figure 9-14.
Xiphoid process	Inferior tip of the sternum. Palpate at the distal end of the sternum. See Figure 9-15.
Costovertebral joints	Articulation of the vertebra and ribs. Cannot be palpated.
Sternocostal joints	Articulation of the sternum and ribs. Difficult to distinguish.
Costal cartilage	Cartilage joining ribs and sternum. Difficult to distinguish.

2. Palpation of muscles:

   A. Locate the following muscles on the skeleton and anatomical models, and on at least one partner.

      • The information needed to palpate each muscle is provided in the following tables.

      • The position described for locating the muscle on your partner is usually the manual muscle test position for a fair or better grade of muscle strength.

      • Not all origins, insertions, and muscle bellies can be palpated on your partner.

   B. On the skeleton, locate the origin and insertion of each muscle.

      • Place the ends of a rubber band at the origin and insertion of the muscle, making the band taut. Note the location of the muscle in relation to the joints it crosses.

Supine Position

DIAPHRAGM:	Located deep, separates thoracic and abdominal cavities

FIGURE 16-5 Palpating the diaphragm.

Position of person:	Quiet breathing
Origin:	Xiphoid process, lower six ribs, upper lumbar vertebrae
Insertion:	Central tendon
Line of pull:	Diagonal
Muscle action:	Inspiration
Observe:	Chest and abdomen rise
Palpate:	Palpate by curling your fingers under the inferior edge of the rib cage bilaterally. You may not feel the contraction of the diaphragm but may feel other tissues being pushed out as the diaphragm contracts. Alternatively, place your hand over the upper abdomen, noting the rise and fall of the abdomen as the person breathes.
Instructions to person:	Breathe in and out at your normal rate.
EXTERNAL INTERCOSTALS:	Located between ribs

FIGURE 16-6 Palpating the external intercostals.

Position of person:	Quiet breathing
Origin:	Rib above
Insertion:	Rib below
Line of pull:	Diagonal
Muscle action:	Elevate ribs
Palpate:	Between adjacent ribs on the side of the rib cage, inferior to the pectoralis major muscle attachments
Instructions to person:	Breathe in and out at your normal rate.
INTERNAL INTERCOSTALS:	Located between ribs deep to external intercostals
Position of person:	Quiet breathing
Origin:	Rib below
Insertion:	Rib above
Line of pull:	Diagonal
Muscle action:	Depress ribs
Palpate:	Between adjacent ribs; difficult because they are deep muscles and difficult to distinguish from the external intercostals
Instructions to person:	Breathe in and out at your normal rate.

3. Observe the amount of motion available as the rib cage moves during quiet respiration and deep respiration.

   A. Place the palm and fingers of one hand over your partner's xiphoid process and the other hand over the spinous process of the T8 through T10 vertebrae. Note the extent of chest expansion in the anterior-posterior (A-P) direction during quiet breathing.

   • Ask your partner to inhale deeply and exhale fully several times slowly and note extent of chest expansion in the A-P direction.

B. Place your hands over the eighth to tenth ribs bilaterally in the midaxillary line. Note the extent of chest expansion in the transverse direction during quiet breathing.

- Ask your partner to inhale deeply and exhale fully several times slowly, and note the extent of chest expansion in the transverse direction.

C. Use a tape measure to measure the difference in rib cage circumference.

- To determine any differences based on gender, age, and smoker/nonsmoker status, compare the measurements of classmates who volunteer to participate.

4. Using two pencils and the skeleton, align both pencils, with lead end pointing up, on the anterior of the rib cage in the direction of the muscle fibers of the external intercostal muscles. Move one pencil around the ribs to the posterior rib cage. Compare the alignment of the pencils.

A. Anteriorly, is the eraser end pointing medially or laterally?

B. Posteriorly, is the eraser end pointing medially or laterally?

C. Why does the angle appear to change?

5. Palpate your partner's upper trapezius and sternocleidomastoid muscles (1) during quiet breathing and (2) during deep breathing. Is there any difference? Why?

6. With your partner in the supine position, head resting on a small pillow and legs supported so the low back is relaxed:

A. Place one hand on your partner's chest and one hand on the stomach. During quiet breathing, what movements do you see and feel?

1) What type of breathing is occurring if the hand on the stomach moves and the hand on the chest moves very little? _____

2) What type of breathing is occurring if the hand on the chest moves the most?

B. Palpate your partner's upper and lower rib cage during quiet breathing. What movement do you see and feel?

C. Repeat A and B as your partner takes deep breaths. Describe any changes and explain why they occur.

D. Palpate your partner's rib cage and abdomen as your partner coughs, sneezes, and talks. Compare and contrast the movements of the rib cage and abdomen during these maneuvers and to movements during quiet respiration.

7. Using proper body mechanics, lift your lab manual off a treatment table. Using proper body mechanics, lift a backpack filled with books or weights. Observe differences in breathing.

8. With your partner lying supine, ask her or him to flex head and neck while you palpate your partner's abdomen.

A. Repeat and ask your partner to not use any abdominal muscles. Compare the two experiences.

B. What is the function of the abdominals when lifting the head?

C. How does this relate to breathing?

■ ■ ■ Post-Lab Questions

Student's Name _____

Date Due _____

After you have completed the worksheets and lab activities, answer the following questions without using your book or notes. When finished, check your answers.

1. List the bones of the rib cage.

   _____

   _____

2. List the joints of the rib cage.

   _____

   _____

3. List the motions of the rib cage.

   _____

   _____

4. List the muscles of quiet respiration.

   _____

   _____

   _____

5. What is the innervation of the prime movers for respiration?

   _____

   _____

6. Cervical spinal cord lesions can interfere with the ability of individuals to breathe on their own. Above what level of spinal cord lesion does an individual require assistance of a ventilator to breathe?

   _____

7. Describe the mechanics of quiet respiration by the phases of respiration.

   _____

   _____

   _____

   _____

8. During quiet inspiration, the diaphragm is contacting:

   _____ Concentrically _____ Eccentrically
   _____ Isometrically

9. The ribs can be described by their attachments and locations.

   A. Which ribs attach to the sternum by way of their own individual costal cartilage? _____

   B. Which ribs attach to the sternum by way of a common costal cartilage? _____

   C. Which ribs attach only to the vertebral column? _____

   D. Which rib lies deep to the superior angle of the scapula? _____

   E. Which rib lies deep to the inferior angle of the scapula? _____

10. What positions of the upper extremities do sprinters often assume immediately after a race? Why?

    _____

    _____

    _____

11. What is the function of the upper trapezius during respiration by persons with chronic obstructive respiratory disease?

    _____

    _____

12. Persons with chronic obstructive respiratory disease often sit leaning forward propped on their arms. How does this posture contribute to ease of respiration?

    _____

    _____

13. Why might a person with emphysema lean with the forearms on the handgrip of a grocery cart while walking through a grocery store?

_____

_____

_____

_____

_____

_____

14. In many sports, as athletes perform a strenuous activity, such as during the lift for a power lifter, throwing the shot put, or returning a serve, they can be heard to exhale. Why is this advantageous?

_____

Pelvic Girdle

■ ■ ■ Pre-Lab Worksheets

Student's Name _____

Date Due _____

Complete the following questions prior to the lab class.

1. Match the following terms with the appropriate definition:

_____ False pelvis	A. Sacral base moves anteriorly and inferiorly.
_____ Pelvic inlet	B. A line from the tip of the coccyx to the inferior surface of the pubic symphysis
_____ Pelvic outlet	C. Occurs when the base of the sacrum moves posteriorly and superiorly
_____ True pelvis	D. Bony area between the iliac crests and superior to the pelvic inlet
_____ Pelvic cavity	E. Located between the inlet and the outlet of the pelvis
_____ Nutation	F. Located between the sacral promontory and superior border of symphysis pubis
_____ Counternutation	G. Forms the birth canal

2. On Figures 17-1A, B, and C, label the following bones, landmarks, and joints of the pelvic girdle:

BONES and LANDMARKS

SACRUM: Base   Superior   Auricular
                          articular   surface
                          process

            Posterior   Ala
            foramina

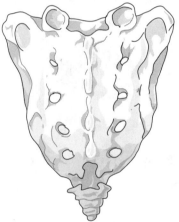

FIGURE 17-1A Landmarks of the posterior sacrum.

HIP BONES: Ilium   Ischium   Pubis

LANDMARKS:	Iliac crest	Greater sciatic notch	Ischial tuberosity
	PSIS	PIIS	Ischial body
	Ischial spine	ASIS	Lesser sciatic notch
	AIIS	Acetabulum	Superior ramus
	Body of pubis	Inferior ramus	

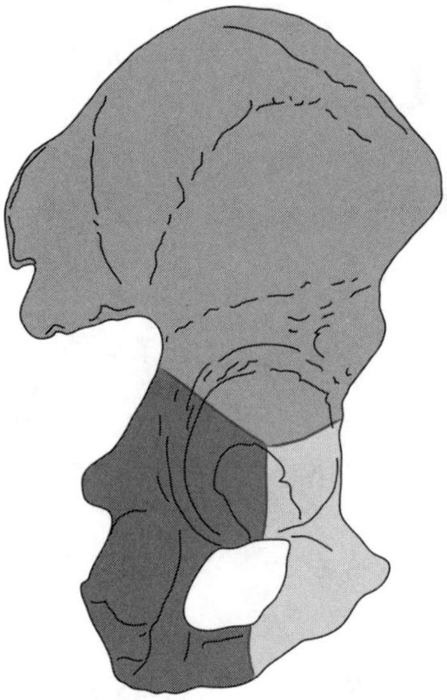

JOINTS OF THE PELVIC GIRDLE:	Sacroiliac joints	Symphysis pubis	Lumbosacral joint

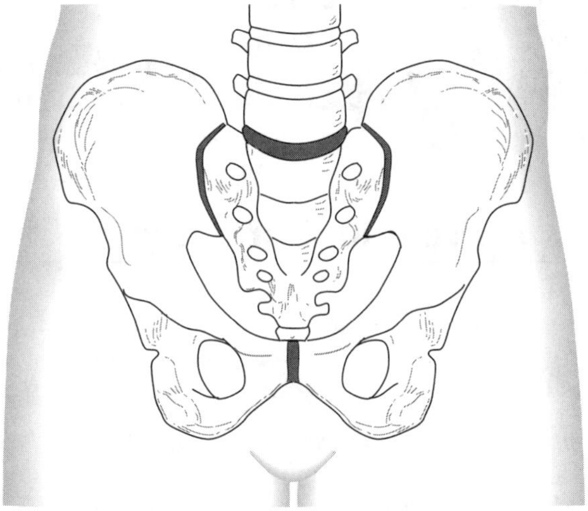

FIGURE 17-1C Joints of the pelvis.

FIGURE 17-1B Bones, landmarks of the lateral pelvis.

3. On Figures 17-2A, B, and C, label the following ligaments:

Anterior sacroiliac ligament	Inguinal ligament
Short posterior sacroiliac ligament	Long posterior sacroiliac ligament
Sacrotuberous ligament	Sacrospinous ligament
Iliolumbar ligament	Superior pubic ligament
Inferior pubic ligament	Lumbosacral ligament

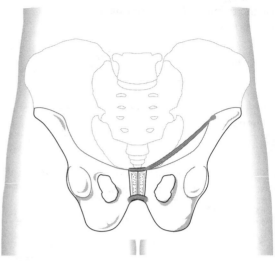

FIGURE 17-2C Ligaments of the pubic symphysis.

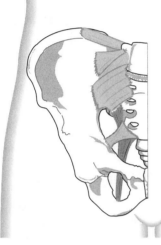

FIGURE 17-2A Ligaments of the anterior pelvis.

4. Indicate which of the following statements are true of the female pelvis and which are true of the male pelvis by placing an F or M, respectively, by the statement.

_____	Heart-shaped pelvic cavity opening	_____	Rounded pelvic cavity opening
_____	Short pelvic cavity	_____	Funnel-shaped pelvic cavity
_____	Short sacrum	_____	Ischial tuberosities far apart

5. For the following joint, indicate which motions are available, in which plane the motion occurs, and about which axis the motion occurs.

Joint	Motions	Plane	Axis
Sacroiliac			

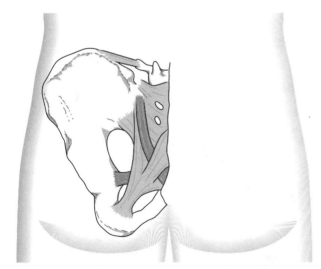

FIGURE 17-2B Ligaments of the posterior pelvis.

6. List the trunk and hip motions that accompany SI joint motions.

SI Motion	Trunk	Hip
Nutation (flexion)		
Counternutation (extension)		

7. Review previous chapters and list the anterior trunk muscles that attach to the pelvis.

_____

_____

8. Review previous chapters and list the posterior trunk and upper extremity muscles that attach to the pelvis.

_____

_____

9. List three motions of the pelvis.

_____

_____

■ ■ ■ Lab Activities

Student's Name _____

Date Due _____

1. Palpation of bones and landmarks:

   - Locate the following structures on bones or skeleton, and palpate on your partner when possible.
   - The reference position is the anatomical position.
   - Not all structures can be palpated on your partner.

Sacrum

Base	Superior surface of S1. Cannot be palpated.
Promontory	Ridge projecting along the anterior edge of the body of S1. Cannot be palpated.
Superior articular process	Located posteriorly on the base, it articulates with the inferior articular process of L5. Cannot be palpated.
Ala	Lateral flared wings that are actually fused transverse processes. Cannot be palpated.
Foramina	Four pair located on the anterior and dorsal surfaces lateral to midline. They serve as the exit for the anterior and posterior divisions of the sacral nerves. The anterior foramina are larger and cannot be palpated. Difficult to palpate on posterior surface.
Auricular surface	Located on the lateral surface of the sacrum and articulates with the ilium. Cannot be palpated.
Pelvic surface	Concave anterior surface. Cannot be palpated.

Ilium

Tuberosity	Large roughened area between the posterior portion of the iliac crest and the auricular surface. It is the attachment for the interosseous ligament. Cannot be palpated.
Auricular surface	The articular surface of the ilium with the sacrum. Located inferior and anterior to the iliac tuberosity. Cannot be palpated.
Iliac crest	Superior margin of ilium extending from the ASIS to the PSIS. Iliac crests appear to be located more superiorly in men than women. Palpate by placing your hand on the top margin of the pelvis (place your hands on your hips). **FIGURE 17-3** Palpating the iliac crest.
Greater sciatic notch	Formed by the ilium superiorly and the ilium and ischium inferiorly. Cannot be palpated.
Greater sciatic foramen	Formed from the greater sciatic notch by ligamentous attachments. Cannot be palpated.

Continued

Ilium—Cont'd

Posterior superior iliac spine (PSIS)	Posterior projection of the iliac crest. It is the attachment for the posterior sacroiliac ligaments. Palpate by placing your hand on the iliac crest and moving posterior and medially to the first protuberance. A "dimple" is usually observable over the PSIS. **FIGURE 17-4** Palpating the posterior superior iliac spine (PSIS).
Posterior inferior iliac spine (PIIS)	Protuberance located inferior to the PSIS. It is the attachment for the sacrotuberous ligament. Palpate by moving inferiorly from the PSIS.

Ischium

Body	Makes up the entire ischium superior to the tuberosity. Cannot be palpated.
Lesser sciatic notch	Smaller cavity located on the posterior body between the greater sciatic notch and the ischial tuberosity. Cannot be palpated.
Spine	Located on the posterior body and between the greater sciatic and lesser sciatic notches. Attachment for the sacrospinous ligament. Cannot be palpated.
Tuberosity	The blunt, rough projection on the inferior part of the body. Palpate by having your partner flex at the trunk. Move your fingers up the posterior thigh to the large protuberance located slightly medial on the inferior buttock.

FIGURE 17-5 Palpating the ischial tuberosity.

Ramus	Extends anteriorly from the body to connect with the inferior ramus of the pubis; it is the attachment for the adductor magnus, obturator externus, and obturator internus. Palpation is usually not possible.

Pubis

Body	Main portion of the pubic bone. Palpation is difficult.
Superior ramus	Superior projection of the pubic body. Palpation is easier on self; palpate just lateral to the midline.
Inferior ramus	Inferior projection of the pubic body. It is the attachment for the inferior pubic ligament. Cannot be palpated.
Tubercle	Projects anteriorly on the superior ramus near the midline. It is the attachment for the superior pubic ligament. Not easily palpated.
Symphysis pubis	Cartilaginous joint connecting the bodies of the two pubic bones at the anterior midline. Palpation is usually not performed.

2. Palpation of joints and ligaments

- Locate the following structures on a skeleton, and palpate on your partner when possible.

Ligament	Location	Function
Anterior sacroiliac	Attaches on the anterior surface connecting the ala and pelvic surface of the sacrum to the auricular surface of the ilium	Holds the anterior portion of the joint. Connects the tuberosities together.
Interosseous sacroiliac	Attaches to the tuberosities of the ilium to the sacrum	Connects the tuberosities of the ilium to the sacrum
Short posterior sacroiliac	Attaches to the ilium and the upper portion of the sacrum on the dorsal surface	Prevents forward movement of the sacrum
Long posterior sacroiliac	Attaches to the posterior superior iliac, spine, and the lower portion of the sacrum	Prevents downward movement of the sacrum
Sacrotuberous	Attaches to the posterior lateral side of the sacrum inferior to the auricular surface, the coccyx, and the ischial tuberosity	An attachment for the gluteus maximus, and prevents forward rotation of the sacrum
Sacrospinous	Attaches to the lower, lateral sacrum and coccyx on the posterior side and the spine of the ischium	With the sacrotuberous, makes the sciatic notch into a foramen
Iliolumbar	Attaches to the transverse process of L5 and the posterior portion of the iliac crest	Limits the rotation of L5 on S1 and assists the articular processes in preventing L5 from moving anteriorly on S1
Superior pubic	Attaches to the pubic tubercles on each side of the body	Strengthens the superior and anterior portions of the pubic symphysis
Inferior pubic	Attaches between the inferior pubic rami	Strengthens the inferior portion of the pubic symphysis
Lumbosacral	Attaches on the transverse process of L5 and the ala of the sacrum	Reinforces the sacroiliac ligaments

3. Perform the motions of the pelvis (lateral, anterior, and posterior tilt, and rotation).

   A. Perform a motion and then your partner names the motion you performed.

   B. Your partner states a motion and then you perform that motion.

4. As you perform the following pelvic motions, what happens at the lumbar spine and hips?

Pelvic Motion	Lumbar Spine	Hips
Anterior pelvic tilt		
Posterior pelvic tilt		
Lateral pelvic tilt to the right		

5. For each of the motions of the pelvis:

A. Place your open left hand in the correct orientation to represent the plane of a motion.

B. Place your right index finger to indicate the axis of that motion.

C. Enter the plane and axis for each motion in the following table.

Pelvic Motions	Plane	Axis
Anterior/posterior tilt		
Lateral tilt		
Rotation		

6. Using a goniometer, examine the lumbosacral angle of your partner as your partner stands in her or his normal posture and then performs anterior and posterior pelvic tilts.

- Place the axis of the goniometer at the lumbosacral joint.

- Arrange one arm to project posteriorly and horizontal to the floor.

- Place the other arm of the goniometer vertically and parallel to the sacrum.

- Adjust the alignment of the arms as your partner moves, keeping one arm horizontal and the other parallel to the sacrum.

- Note the angle formed in each position: natural, anterior tilt, and posterior tilt.

A. Approximately what is your partner's lumbosacral angle when in:

1) Normal posture: _____

2) Anterior tilt: _____

3) Posterior tilt: _____

B. How do the measurements you obtained compare to the normal angle of approximately 30 degrees?

_____

7. A. Sit in front of your standing partner. Place your thumbs on your partner's anterior superior iliac spines (ASIS).

1) Are they level? _____ Yes _____ No

Which is high? _____ Right _____ Left

2) When your partner lifts the left foot off the floor without flexing the hip or knee (i.e., performs hip hiking), describe what happens to the iliac crest.

_____

3) What happens to the pelvis when your partner shifts weight to the right leg and lifts the left foot off the floor by flexing the knee?

_____

4) Observe as your partner takes one step forward with the left foot.

What pelvic motion is produced? _____

What motion, other than hyperextension, occurs at the right hip? _____

B. Sit facing one side of your partner who is standing. Place one index finger on your partner's ASIS and your other index finger on your partner's posterior superior iliac spine (PSIS).

1) Are they level? _____ Yes _____ No

Which is high? _____ ASIS _____ PSIS

2) What happens when your partner performs an anterior pelvic tilt?

_____

3) What happens when your partner performs a posterior pelvic tilt?

_____

8. Pelvic motions are produced by force couples consisting of muscles on opposite sides of the pelvis. Examine the skeleton and perform the motions to answer the following. Circle the correct answers.

A. When contracting concentrically, which trunk muscles produce an anterior pelvic tilt?

Extensors   Flexors

B. Which hip muscles would be in a position to assist the trunk muscles to produce an anterior pelvic tilt?

Extensors   Flexors   Abductors   Adductors

C. When contracting concentrically, which trunk muscles produce a posterior pelvic tilt?

Extensors   Flexors

D. Which hip muscles would be in a position to assist the trunk muscles to produce a posterior pelvic tilt?

Extensors   Flexors   Abductors   Adductors

E. Which trunk muscles produce a right lateral pelvic tilt?

Left trunk flexors   Right trunk flexors

F. Which hip muscles would be in a position to assist the trunk muscles to control a lateral pelvic tilt to the right (right side lower than left)?

Extensors   Flexors
Right abductors   Left abductors

G. When performing a lateral pelvic tilt, the hip muscles are moving the
_____ distal insertion toward the proximal insertion.

_____ proximal insertion toward the distal insertion.

9. When standing, how does performing an anterior or posterior tilt of the pelvis affect the lumbar curves of the spine?

Pelvic Tilt	Lumbar Curves
Anterior	
Posterior	

10. What is the effect on the position of the pelvis and lumbar spine in the following positions and activities?

A. Sitting on a low stool:

_____

_____

B. Sitting on a high stool so that your feet only barely touch the floor:

_____

_____

C. While sitting on the low stool, catch a ball and throw it to hit a specific target. What effect did the sitting position have on your ability to toss and catch a ball?

_____

_____

D. Repeat part C while sitting on the high stool. What effect did this sitting position have on your ability to toss and catch the ball?

_____

_____

E. Repeat part C while sitting on a stool that allows you to sit with your feet supported and your thighs parallel to the floor. What effect did this sitting position have on your ability to toss and catch the ball?

_____

_____

■ ■ ■ Post-Lab Questions

Student's Name _____

Date Due _____

After you have completed the worksheets and lab activities, answer the following questions without using your book or notes. When finished, check your answers.

1. List the pelvic motions:

   _____

2. Does Figure 17-6 illustrate an anterior or posterior tilt? _____

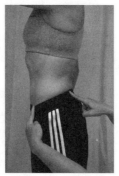

FIGURE 17-6 Pelvic tilt.

3. Describe the force couples that produce:

   A. An anterior pelvic tilt:

   _____

   B. A posterior pelvic tilt:

   _____

   C. A lateral pelvic hike:

   _____

4. What motion occurs at the hip as the following are performed?

   A. Anterior pelvic tilt:

   _____

   B. Posterior pelvic tilt:

   _____

   C. Pelvic rotation to the right (forward):

   _____

5. What muscle, by itself, produces hip hiking when a person is supine?

   _____

6. Shortness of which muscle groups will produce the following postures?

   A. Anterior pelvic tilt:

   _____

   B. Posterior pelvic tilt:

   _____

   C. In standing on the left, a lateral pelvic tilt to the right:

   _____

   _____

7. A. In late stages of pregnancy, many women assume what position of the pelvis? Why?

   _____ Anterior tilt   _____ Posterior tilt

   _____

   B. What posture does the upper body assume to compensate for the pelvic position?

   _____

Clinical Kinesiology and Anatomy of the Lower Extremities

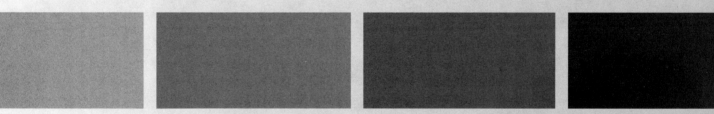

Hip Joint

■ ■ ■ Pre-Lab Worksheets

Student's Name _____

Date Due _____

Complete the following questions prior to the lab class.

1. Match the following terms with their descriptors.

   A.

   _____ Coxa valgus   A. 125°

   _____ Coxa varus   B. Greater than 130°

   _____ Angle of inclination C. Less than 125°

   B.

   _____ Angel of torsion   A. Less than 15°

   _____ Anteversion   B. 15°–25°

   _____ Retroversion   C. Greater than 25°

2. On Figures 18-1, 18-2, and 18-3, label the following hip bones and landmarks. Review the landmarks of the pelvis in Chapter 17.

HIP BONES: Ilium   Pubis   Ischium

LANDMARKS:	Iliac crest	Anterior superior iliac spine	Anterior inferior iliac spine
	Acetabulum	Superior ramus	Body of pubis
	Inferior ramus	Posterior superior iliac spine	Posterior inferior iliac spine
	Greater sciatic notch	Ischial spine	Lesser sciatic notch
	Body of ischium	Obturator foramen	Ischial tuberosity
	Ramus		

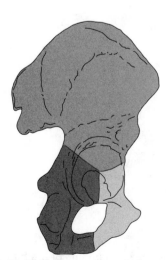

FIGURE 18-1 Right hip bone, lateral view.

FEMUR:

Head	Neck	Body
	Greater trochanter	Lesser trochanter
	Medial condyle	Lateral condyle
	Medial epicondyle	Lateral epicondyle
	Linea aspera	Pectineal line
	Adductor tubercle	

TIBIA: Tibial tuberosity

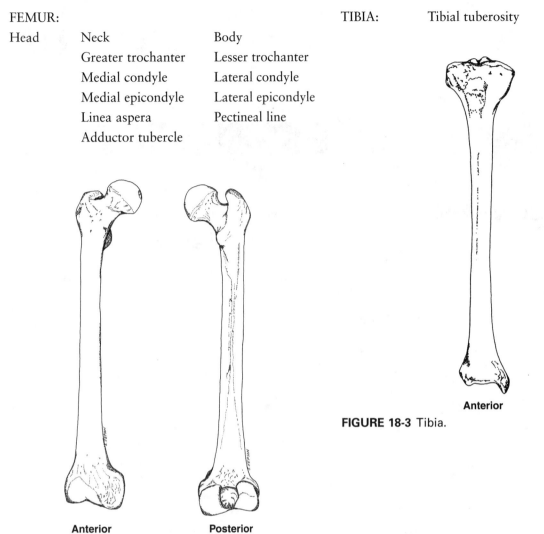

FIGURE 18-2 Femur.

Anterior   Posterior

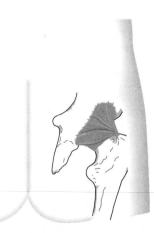

Anterior

FIGURE 18-3 Tibia.

3. On Figures 18-4 and 18-5, label the following structures:

A. Iliofemoral ligament   Pubofemoral ligament
   Ischiofemoral ligament

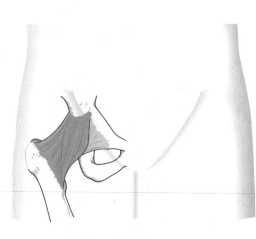

Anterior   Posterior

FIGURE 18-4 Ligaments of the hip.

B. Iliotibial band

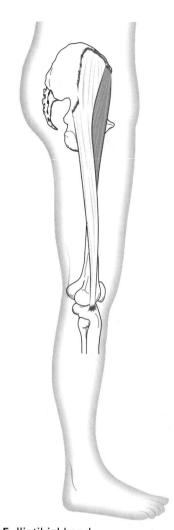

FIGURE 18-5 Iliotibial band.

4. On Figures 18-6 through 18-10:

A. Label the origin and insertion of the muscles listed.

B. Join the origin and insertion to show the line of pull.

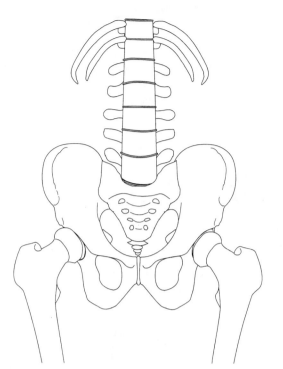

FIGURE 18-6 Iliopsoas and pectineus.

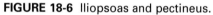

FIGURE 18-7 Rectus femoris, and sartorius.

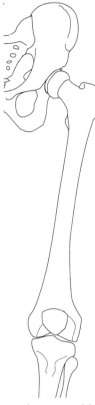

FIGURE 18-8 Adductor longus, adductor brevis, adductor magnus, and gracilis.

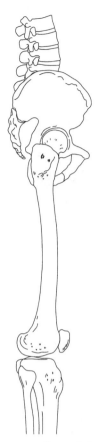

FIGURE 18-10 Gluteus medius, gluteus minimus, and tensor fascia latae.

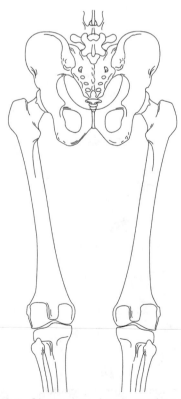

FIGURE 18-9 Gluteus maximus, semimembranosus, semitendinosus, and biceps femoris.

5. For the hip joint, give the following information:

Joint	Shape	Degrees of Freedom	Motions	Plane	Axis
Hip					

6. At the hip joint, identify which surface is concave and which is convex.

Joint	Concave	Convex
Hip		

7. For the hip joint, provide the close-packed position and the loose-packed position (refer to Chapter 4, Table 4-4 for descriptions).

Joint	Close-Packed	Loose-Packed
Hip		

8. For the hip joint, indicate the normal end feel (refer to Chapter 4, Table 4-1 for descriptions).

_____ Bony _____ Soft tissue stretch
_____ Soft tissue approximation

9. Analyze the activity of the leg being moved out to the side while in the supine position.

A. Which joint motion is being analyzed?

_____

B. Identify the "axis" of the motion:

_____

C. Would gravity cause the movement?

_____

D. Is the "resistance" to the movement a muscle or the weight of the leg? _____

E. Which major muscle group is the agonist?

_____

F. Is the agonist performing a concentric or an eccentric contraction? _____

G. Is this an open or closed kinetic chain activity?

_____

10. The hip muscles can be divided into four major groups by location: anterior, posterior, medial, and lateral. Identify the main action of each location and major innervation by location.

Location	Action	Innervation
Anterior		
Medial		
Posterior		
Lateral		

11. Match the following ligaments and structures to their function.

_____ Joint capsule

_____ Iliofemoral ligament

_____ Pubofemoral ligament

_____ Ischiofemoral ligament

_____ Ligamentum teres

_____ Acetabular labrum

_____ Inguinal ligament

_____ Iliotibial band

A. Reinforces hip joint capsule anteriorly

B. Contains blood vessels to the femoral head

C. Encases head and neck of femur

D. Limits abduction of hip joint

E. Insertion for gluteus maximus and tensor fascia latae

F. Assists to hold head of femur in acetabulum

G. Reinforces hip joint capsule posteriorly

H. Landmark denoting separation of trunk from the leg

12. For each hip motion listed, check the muscle(s) that are major contributors to that action.

Motion	Iliopsoas	Rectus Femoris	Sartorius	Pectineus	Adductor Magnus	Adductor Longus	Adductor Brevis	Gracilis
Flexion								
Extension								
Hyperextension								
Abduction								
Adduction								
Medial rotation								
Lateral rotation								

Motion	Gluteus Maximus	Gluteus Medius	Gluteus Minimus	Semimembranosus	Semitendinosus	Biceps Femoris	Tensor Fascia Latae	Deep Rotator Group
Flexion								
Extension								
Hyperextension								
Abduction								
Adduction								
Medial rotation								
Lateral rotation								

■ ■ ■ Lab Activities

Student's Name _____

Date Due _____

1. Palpation of joints, ligaments, and other structures:
   - Locate on bones and skeleton, and palpate when possible.
   - The reference position is the anatomical position.
   - Not all structures are palpable on your partner.
   - Review Chapter 17 for structures on the ischium and pubis.

Ilium

Iliac fossa	Large, smooth, concave area on the internal surface; attachment for the iliopsoas muscle. It cannot be palpated because of the iliopsoas muscle and abdominal contents. From just above the ASIS on the iliac crest, however, you may be able to roll your fingers over into the fossa area.
Iliac crest	Superior margin of ilium extending from the ASIS to the PSIS. Iliac crests appear to be located more superiorly in men than women. Palpate by placing your hand on the top margin of the pelvis. See Figure 17-3.
Anterior superior iliac spine (ASIS)	The projection on the anterior end of the iliac crest; attachment for the tensor fascia latae, sartorius, and inguinal ligament. Palpate by moving to the anterior-most point of the iliac crest.

FIGURE 18-11 Palpating the ASIS.

Anterior inferior iliac spine (AIIS)	The projection just inferior to the ASIS; attachment for the rectus femoris. Can be difficult to palpate because it is deep to muscle.
Posterior superior iliac spine (PSIS)	Posterior projection of the iliac crest. It is the attachment for the posterior sacroiliac ligaments. Palpate by placing your hand on the iliac crest and moving posterior and medially to the first protuberance. A "dimple" is usually observable over the PSIS. See Figure 17-4.
Posterior inferior iliac spine (PIIS)	Protuberance located inferior to the PSIS. It is the attachment for the sacrotuberous ligament. Palpate by moving inferiorly from the PSIS.

Femur

Head	Rounded portion on the proximal medial border of the femur; articulates with the acetabulum. Cannot be palpated.
Neck	Narrow portion located between the head and the trochanters. Cannot be palpated.
Greater trochanter	Large protuberance located on the proximal lateral aspect between the neck and the body of the femur. It is the attachment for the gluteus medius and minimus, and for most deep rotators. Easily palpated by placing your fingers on the proximal lateral aspect of the femur; as the femur is rotated, the greater trochanter can be felt as it rolls under your fingers.

FIGURE 18-12 Palpating the greater trochanter.

Lesser trochanter	Smaller protuberance located slightly posteriorly on the proximal, medial femur distal to the greater trochanter; attachment for the iliopsoas. Palpation is usually not possible.

Continued

Femur—Cont'd

Shaft or body	Long cylindrical portion, bowed slightly anteriorly; attachment for the hamstrings and quadriceps. Palpation is usually not possible.
Medial condyle	Rounded portion on the distal medial end just proximal to the knee joint. With knee flexed and muscle relaxed, palpate on the medial side. It is being palpated by the examiner's left hand. **FIGURE 18-13** Palpating the medial and lateral condyles.
Lateral condyle	Rounded portion on the distal lateral end just proximal to the knee joint. With the knee flexed and the muscle relaxed, palpate on the lateral side. In Figure 18-13, it is being palpated by the examiner's right hand.
Medial epicondyle	Projection proximal to the medial condyle. With the knee flexed, move your fingers medially to the inside of the knee and proximal to the medial condyle.
Lateral epicondyle	Projection proximal to the lateral condyle. With the knee flexed, move your fingers laterally to the outside of the knee and proximal to the lateral condyle.
Adductor tubercle	Small projection proximal to the medial epicondyle. It is the attachment for a portion of the adductor magnus. With the knee extended, find the spot just superior to the medial epicondyle. Move your fingers back and forth across the adductor magnus tendon. Usually tender to touch.

Linea aspera	Prominent longitudinal ridge or crest running most of the length of the posterior side. Cannot be palpated.
Patellar surface	Located on the distal anterior surface between the condyles. Articulates with the posterior surface of the patella. The patellar surface can be palpated when the knee is fully flexed and the patella has moved distally. Place your fingers just above the superior border of the patella. Do not move your fingers as you flex the knee. **FIGURE 18-14** Patellar surface.

Tibia

Tibial tuberosity	Large projection located on the proximal anterior midline of the tibia; attachment for the patellar tendon. Because this projection is often visually evident, palpation is easy. With the knee flexed and the muscle relaxed, palpate by moving distally from the patella along the patellar tendon to the insertion. **FIGURE 18-15** Palpating the tibial tuberosity.

Ligaments and Other Structures

Iliofemoral ligament, or "Y" ligament	Crosses the joint anteriorly from the AIIS to the intertrochanteric line of the femur—a line between the greater and lesser trochanters. Because the ligament splits before inserting on the femur, it resembles the letter Y. Cannot be palpated.
Pubofemoral ligament	Crosses the hip on the medial inferior side, passing posteriorly and inferiorly from the medial aspect of the acetabular rim and superior ramus of the pubis to the neck of the femur. Cannot be palpated.
Ischiofemoral ligament	Crosses the hip on the posterior side, passing laterally and proximally from the ischial portion of the acetabulum to the femoral neck. Cannot be palpated.
Ligamentum teres	A small intercapsular ligament that attaches to the acetabulum and the fovea of the femoral head. Cannot be palpated.
Acetabular labrum	Located around the rim of the acetabulum, thereby increasing the depth of the acetabulum and surrounding the head of the femur, contributes to holding the head in the acetabulum. Cannot be palpated.
Inguinal ligament	Located on the anterior surface, it serves as the boundary between the trunk and the lower extremity. With the knees and hips slightly flexed and relaxed (support on a bolster), palpate the ASIS and then move your fingers diagonally downward to the symphysis pubis (in the bend of the hip). Move your fingers back and forth across the ligament. Just distal to this, palpate the femoral pulse as the femoral artery and vein pass under it.
Iliotibial band or tract (IT band)	Located on the lateral aspect of the thigh, attaching to the anterior portion of the iliac crest and the proximal anterior lateral tibia. Attachment for the gluteus maximus and tensor fascia latae. Palpate the tendon of the biceps

femoris located posterior and proximal to the knee. Palpate the IT band lateral to the biceps femoris tendon. Move your fingers side to side across the IT band. Extending and adducting the hip may cause the IT band to be more prominent on the lateral side of the thigh.

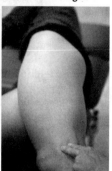

FIGURE 18-16 Palpating the IT band.

2. Palpation of muscles:

A. Locate the following muscles on the skeleton and anatomical models, and on at least one partner.

- The information needed to palpate each muscle is provided in the following tables.
- The position described for locating the muscle on your partner is usually the manual muscle test position for a fair or better grade of muscle strength.
- Not all origins, insertions, and muscle bellies can be palpated on your partner.

B. On the skeleton, locate the origin and insertion of each muscle.

- Place the ends of a rubber band at the origin and insertion of the muscle, making the band taut. Note the location of the muscle in relation to the joints it crosses.
- When possible, move the skeleton to perform the muscle's motion and observe how the band becomes less taut, similar to the change in length as it performs a concentric contraction.

Sitting Position

ILIOPSOAS:	A deep muscle located on the anterior aspect of the hip joint

FIGURE 18-17 Palpating the iliopsoas.

Position of person:	Sitting with hip and knee in about 90° of flexion and neutral alignment
Origin:	Anterior surface of the iliac fossa, the anterior and lateral surfaces of the vertebral bodies and the transverse processes of T12–L5
Insertion:	Lesser trochanter of the femur
Line of pull:	Vertical on the anterior surface of the hip joint
Muscle action:	Hip flexion
Palpate:	At the midline in the "bend" of the hip, distal to the inguinal ligament
Instructions to person:	Flex your hip and lift your thigh straight up and off the table.

RECTUS FEMORIS:	A superficial muscle located on the anterior thigh. This muscle is one part of the quadriceps muscle.

FIGURE 18-18 Palpating the rectus femoris.

Position of person:	Sitting with hip and knee in about 90° of flexion and neutral alignment
Origin:	Anterior inferior iliac spine
Insertion:	Tibial tuberosity via the patellar tendon
Line of pull:	Vertical on the anterior surface of the hip joint
Muscle action:	Hip flexion and knee extension
Palpate:	As it crosses anterior to the hip joint lateral to the iliopsoas
Instructions to person:	Flex your hip and lift your thigh straight up and off the table.

SARTORIUS:	A superficial muscle located anterior to the hip joint and medially on the thigh

FIGURE 18-19 Palpating the sartorius.

Position of person:	Sitting with hip and knee in about 90° of flexion and neutral alignment
Origin:	Anterior superior iliac spine
Insertion:	Proximal medial tibia
Line of pull:	Diagonal on the anterior surface of the hip joint
Muscle action:	Simultaneous hip flex, abduction, and lateral rotation and knee flexion
Palpate:	Near the origin or as it crosses diagonally across the thigh
Instructions to person:	Flex your hip and lift your thigh off the table as you place your ankle on the opposite knee.

Side-Lying Position on Same Side as Muscle Being Examined

PECTINEUS:	Located medially and inferior to the hip joint between the adductor longus medially and the iliopsoas laterally
	FIGURE 18-20 Palpating pectineus.
Position of person:	Hip and knee on side being examined in midline, opposite hip and knee flexed with foot on supporting surface or supported in abduction by the examiner
Origin:	Superior ramus of the pubis
Insertion:	Pectineal line of the femur
Line of pull:	Diagonal
Muscle action:	Hip flexion and adduction. The hip lifting the leg off the supporting surface maintains neutral alignment.
Palpate:	On the proximal medial aspect of the thigh
Instructions to person:	Lift your leg up toward the ceiling.
GRACILIS:	A superficial muscle located on the medial thigh
Position of person:	Hip and knee on side being examined in midline, opposite hip and knee flexed with foot on supporting surface
Origin:	Pubis
Insertion:	Proximal anterior medial tibia
Line of pull:	Vertical on the medial surface of the hip joint
Muscle action:	Hip adduction

Palpate:	Palpate on the medial thigh. The adductors are relatively close together and all perform similar motions. Distinguishing between the muscles can be difficult.
Instructions to person:	Lift your leg up toward the ceiling.
ADDUCTOR MAGNUS:	Located on the medial thigh deep to the adductor longus, brevis, and gracilis muscles and anterior to the medial hamstrings
Position of person:	Hip and knee on side being examined in midline, opposite hip and knee flexed with foot on supporting surface
Origin:	Ischial tuberosity and pubis
Insertion:	Entire linea aspera and adductor tubercle
Line of pull:	Diagonal on the medial surface of the hip joint
Muscle action:	Hip adduction
Palpate:	Locate the ischial tuberosity, move slightly forward on the medial aspect of the thigh. Another place to palpate is the distal attachment at the adductor tubercle.
Instructions to person:	Lift your leg up toward the ceiling.
ADDUCTOR LONGUS:	A superficial muscle on the medial thigh
Position of person:	Hip and knee on side being examined in midline, opposite hip and knee flexed with foot on supporting surface
Origin:	Pubis
Insertion:	Middle third of the linea aspera of the femur
Line of pull:	Diagonal on the medial surface of the hip joint
Muscle action:	Hip adduction

Continued

Side-Lying Position on Same Side as Muscle Being Examined—Cont'd

Palpate:	Palpate on the proximal medial thigh. The adductors are relatively close together and all perform the same motion. Distinguishing between the muscles can be difficult.
Instructions to person:	Lift your leg toward the ceiling.
ADDUCTOR BREVIS:	Located deep to the adductor longus muscle
Position of person:	Hip and knee on side being examined in midline, opposite hip and knee flexed with foot on supporting surface
Origin:	Pubis
Insertion:	Pectineal line and proximal linea aspera of the femur
Line of pull:	Diagonal on the medial surface of the hip joint
Muscle action:	Hip adduction
Palpate:	Palpate on the proximal medial thigh. The adductors are relatively close together and all perform the same motion. Distinguishing between the muscles can be difficult.
Instructions to person:	Lift your leg toward the ceiling.

Prone Position

GLUTEUS MAXIMUS:	A superficial muscle on the posterior pelvis

FIGURE 18-21 Palpating the gluteus maximus.

Position of person:	Hip in neutral alignment, knee flexed to about 90°
Origin:	Posterior surfaces of the sacrum and ilium
Insertion:	Posterior femur distal to the greater trochanter and iliotibial band
Line of pull:	Diagonal on the posterior surface of the hip joint
Muscle action:	Hip extension, hyperextension, and lateral rotation. Extend the hip and lift the thigh off the supporting surface, maintaining neutral alignment.
Palpate:	Over the center of the buttocks
Instructions to person:	Lift your leg off the table, keeping your knee bent.
SEMITENDINOSUS:	A superficial muscle on the posterior medial aspect of the thigh

FIGURE 18-22 Palpating the semitendinosus.

Position of person:	Hip extended and knee flexed, and in neutral alignment
Origin:	Ischial tuberosity
Insertion:	Proximal anterior medial tibia
Line of pull:	Vertical on the posterior surface of the hip joint
Muscle action:	Hip extension and knee flexion
Palpate:	Palpate on the posterior medial thigh. The long distal tendon is on the distal medial aspect of the thigh, superficial to the attachment of the semimembranosus.
Instructions to person:	Keep your knee bent and don't let me straighten it.

SEMIMEMBRANOSUS:	Deep to the semitendinosus muscle on the posterior medial thigh

FIGURE 18-23 Palpating the semimembranosus.

Position of person:	Hip and knee extended and in neutral alignment
Origin:	Ischial tuberosity
Insertion:	Posterior surface of the medial condyle of the tibia
Line of pull:	Vertical on the posterior surface of the hip joint
Muscle action:	Hip extension and knee flexion
Palpate:	Palpate on the posterior medial thigh. Distinguishing between the semimembranosus and the semitendinosus can be difficult. The semimembranosus has a broad attachment on the posterior surface of the tibia deep to, and on either side of, the semitendinosus and just proximal to the knee joint.
Instructions to person:	Keep your knee bent and don't let me straighten it.
BICEPS FEMORIS:	A superficial muscle on the posterior lateral thigh.

FIGURE 18-24 Palpating the biceps femoris.

Position of person:	Hip and knee extended and in neutral alignment
Origin:	Long head: Ischial tuberosity Short head: Lateral lip of the linea aspera of the femur
Insertion:	Posterior proximal fibular head
Line of pull:	Vertical on the posterior surface of the hip joint
Muscle action:	Long head: Hip extension and knee flexion Short head: Knee flexion
Palpate:	Palpate on the posterior lateral thigh. The tendon is palpated on the distal lateral thigh at the knee joint.
Instructions to person:	Keep your knee bent and don't let me straighten it.
DEEP ROTATORS:	Deep muscles. Hip rotation is usually examined in sitting position; however, to palpate the muscles, the person is prone.
Position of person:	Hip in extension and neutral rotation and knee in about 90° of flexion
Origin:	Posterior sacrum, ischium, and pubis
Insertion:	Areas of the greater trochanter
Line of pull:	Horizontal on the posterior surface of the hip joint
Muscle action:	Hip lateral rotation
Palpate:	Except for the piriformis, palpation is generally difficult. With one hand, locate the PSIS. With the other hand, locate the coccyx. These landmarks form a T, with the piriformis located along the base of the T. Press on the muscle and have your partner laterally rotate the hip. You may be able to feel the piriformis contracting under the gluteus maximus.
Instructions to person:	Keeping your thigh on the table, roll your leg, moving your foot in.

Side-Lying on Side Opposite Muscle Being Examined

GLUTEUS MEDIUS:	Mostly deep to the gluteus maximus on the posterior and lateral pelvis, except the upper fibers, which are superficial

FIGURE 18-25 Palpating the gluteus medius.

Position of person:	Hip and knee extended in neutral alignment and the lower leg slightly flexed at hip and knee for greater stability
Origin:	Outer surface of the ilium
Insertion:	Lateral surface of the greater trochanter of the femur
Line of pull:	Vertical on the lateral surface of the hip joint
Muscle action:	Abduction of the hip
Palpate:	Palpate on the proximal lateral pelvis and at the insertion on the greater trochanter. Also, palpate in the area just below the iliac crest between the PSIS and the ASIS. May be difficult to distinguish from the gluteus minimus.
Instructions to person:	Lift your top leg to the ceiling.
GLUTEUS MINIMUS:	On the lateral pelvis deep to the gluteus medius
Position of person:	Hip and knee extended in neutral alignment and the lower leg slightly flexed at hip and knee for greater stability
Origin:	Outer surface of the ilium
Insertion:	Anterior surface of the greater trochanter
Line of pull:	Diagonal on the lateral surface of the hip joint

Muscle action:	Hip abduction, medial rotation
Palpate:	Palpate on the lateral aspect of the pelvis and at the insertion. Difficult to distinguish form the gluteus medius.
Instructions to person:	Lift your top leg toward the ceiling.
TENSOR FASCIA LATAE:	A superficial muscle on the proximal anterior lateral thigh between the rectus femoris and the gluteus medius

FIGURE 18-26 Palpating the tensor fascia latae.

Position of person:	Hip and knee extended in neutral alignment and the lower leg slightly flexed at hip and knee for greater stability
Origin:	Anterior superior iliac spine
Insertion:	Lateral condyle of the tibia via the iliotibial band
Line of pull:	Diagonal on the lateral surface of the hip joint
Muscle action:	Combined hip flexion and abduction
Palpate:	Palpate the muscle on the proximal anterior lateral thigh slightly distal and posterior from the ASIS and the iliotibial band on the lateral thigh
Instructions to person:	Lift your top leg toward the ceiling.

3. Perform the motions of the hip joint with your partner.

   A. Perform a motion and have your partner name the motion you performed.

   B. Your partner states a motion and then you perform that motion.

4. Observe the amount of motion available at the hip joint in each plane. For each of the motions, estimate the degrees of motion available by checking the box that *most closely* describes that amount of motion. (Do not measure with a goniometer.)

Motions	0°–45°	46°–90°	91°–135°	136°–180°
Flexion				
Hyperextension				
Abduction				
Adduction				
Medial rotation				
Lateral rotation				

5. Passively move your partner through the available range of motion, making note of the end feel. If possible, repeat with several people. Review worksheet Question 8 for the normal end feel.

   A. Is your partner's end feel consistent with what the end feel is reported to be?

   _____

   B. What structures create the end feels for this joint?

   _____

6. Use a disarticulated skeleton or an anatomical model of the hip joint and apply the rules of joint arthrokinematics and the concave-convex rule to perform the following exercises.

   A. Underline the correct answer.

   The acetabulum is concave/convex.

   The femur is concave/convex.

   B. Move the femur in the acetabulum in all planes of motion.

C. Observe the movement of the femur on the acetabulum. Circle the motions that you observed.

   Roll   Spin   Glide

D. Observe the movement of the distal end of the femur in relation to the movement of the proximal end of the femur as you move the femur in the acetabulum. Does the distal end of the femur move in the _____ same or _____ opposite direction as the proximal end of the femur?

7. For the multijoint muscles of the hip, indicate the positions that simultaneously lengthen or shorten the muscles over all the joints they cross. Move your partner into the lengthened and shortened positions for each muscle.

Muscle	Lengthened Position		Shortened Position	
	Hip	*Knee*	*Hip*	*Knee*
Sartorius				
Semitendinosus				
Semimembranosus				
Biceps femoris— long head				
Rectus femoris				
Gracilis				
Tensor fascia latae				

8. Lying prone, perform hip extension with knee flexion and repeat hip extension with knee extension.

   A. Identify the muscles responsible for hip extension in each position.

   _____

   _____

   B. What position of the knee should a person maintain while performing strengthening exercises of the gluteus maximus muscle? Why?

   _____

   _____

9. **Functional activity analysis:**

In each chapter on the lower extremity, you will be analyzing the activity of moving from sitting to standing, and the reverse motion of moving from standing to sitting. Perform these activities and then analyze how the subject in Figures 18-27 through 18-31 performed those activities.

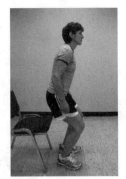

FIGURE 18-30 Midposition—sitting.

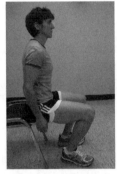

FIGURE 18-27 Starting position for standing up.

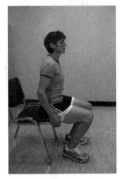

FIGURE 18-31 Assuming sitting.

A. Describe the positions of the hip when the subject is:

1) moving from sitting to standing. _____

_____

2) moving from standing to sitting. _____

_____

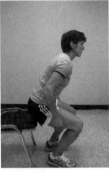

FIGURE 18-28 Initiating standing.

B. Which muscle groups are acting as prime movers while:

1) moving from sitting to standing. _____

_____

2) moving from standing to sitting. _____

_____

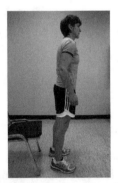

FIGURE 18-29 Ending position—standing. Starting position for sitting down.

C. Describe the type of muscle contraction being used and when:

1) moving from sitting to standing. _____

_____

2) moving from standing to sitting. _____

_____

D. Explain your answers to part C.

1) Moving from sitting to standing. _____

_____

2) Moving from standing to sitting _____

_____

E. Is this an open or closed chain activity?

_____

■ ■ ■ Post-Lab Questions

Student's Name _____

Date Due _____

After you have completed the worksheets and lab activities, answer the following questions without using your book or notes. When finished, check your answers.

1. List the combined joint motions required to put your right ankle on your left knee when you are in a sitting position, and identify the muscle that performs these motions.

   _____

   _____

2. Name the hip muscle that has an attachment on the lumbar spine.

   _____

3. Starting from the anterior midline and proceeding laterally around the knee, list in order the hip muscles that attach below the knee.

   _____

   _____

4. Generally, the following muscle groups share innervation from which peripheral nerves?

   Hamstrings: _____

   Hip flexors: _____

   Hip adductors: _____

5. Applying a deep heat treatment to the posterior lateral pelvis heats the muscles in the area. List the muscles in the order in which they will be heated if the heat penetrates from the most superficial to the deepest muscle.

   _____

   _____

6. The acetabulum is located on the _____ surface of the hip joint.

7. You are to design an exercise program for a person with a problem with her hip. To design the exercise program, you need to know the muscles that attach to the:

   A. Ischial tuberosity. List the muscles that attach to the ischial tuberosity.

      _____

   B. ASIS and AIIS. List the muscles that attach to the ASIS and AIIS.

      ASIS: _____

      AIIS: _____

8. Of the deep rotators of the hip, the piriformis is clinically significant because it can cause nerve compression. Which nerve is in a position to be compressed by the piriformis muscle?

   _____

9. You are assisting family members as they learn to position their thin, frail father who has advanced Parkinson's disease. What bony landmarks must you educate them about for each of the following positions?

   Prone: _____

   Supine: _____

   Side-lying: _____

10. If you placed one finger on the pubic tubercle and your thumb on the ASIS, what structure spans between these two points? _____

11. Lying supine, raise your right lower extremity toward the ceiling.

   A. What motion is occurring at the hip? _____

   B. What is the effect of gravity? _____

   C. What muscles are the agonists? _____

   D. What type of contraction is it? _____

   E. What type of kinetic chain activity is it? _____

   F. Which hip joint surface is convex? _____

   G. What direction is the femoral head surface moving on the acetabular surface in relation to the joint motion? _____

12. For each of the motions available at the hip joint, identify the plane and axis:

Hip Joint	Plane	Axis
Flexion/extension/ hyperextension		
Abduction/adduction		
Medial/lateral rotation		

Knee Joint

■ ■ ■ Pre-Lab Worksheets

Student's Name _____

Date Due _____

Complete the following questions prior to the lab class.

1. The Q angle is often assessed.

    A. Define Q angle:

    _____

    _____

    B. What is the average Q angle? _____

    C. Who has the larger Q angle?

    Men: _____ Women: _____

2. List the muscles that make up the pes anserine.

    _____

    _____

3. Match the following terms that describe the alignment of the lower extremity with the appropriate description.

    _____ Genu valgus   A. Knee joint in more than 0 degrees of extension

    _____ Genu varus   B. Ankle more lateral than normal

    _____ Genu recurvatum   C. Ankle more medial than normal

4. On Figures 19-1 and 19-2, label the following bones, landmarks, and joints:

TIBIA: Intercondylar eminence   Medial condyle
         Lateral condyle   Tibial plateau
         Tibial tuberosity   Medial malleolus
         Crest

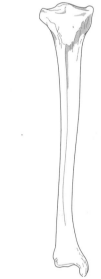

FIGURE 19-1 Right tibia, anterior view.

BONES: Fibula   Tibia   Patella   Calcaneus
JOINTS: Patellofemoral
LAND-   Fibular head   Lateral
MARKS: malleolus

   Patellar
      articular
      surface

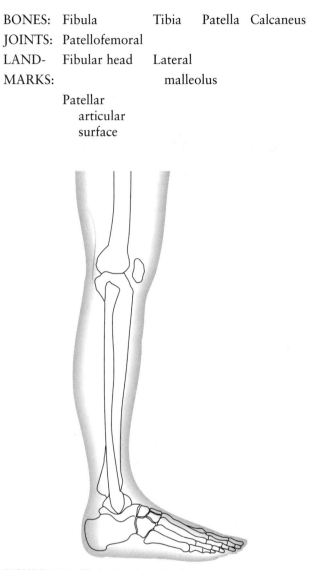

FIGURE 19-2 Right leg, lateral view.

5. On Figure 19-3, label the anterior cruciate and posterior cruciate.

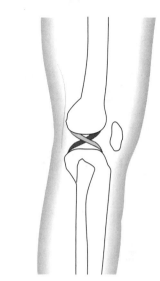

FIGURE 19-3 Knee, lateral view.

6. On Figure 19-4, label the three parts of the pes anserine.

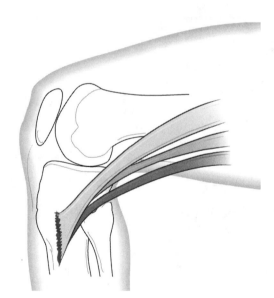

FIGURE19-4 Knee, lateral view.

7. On Figure 19-5, label the following structures of the knee:

Medial collateral ligament	Lateral collateral ligament	Medial meniscus
Lateral meniscus	Lateral tibial condyle	Lateral femoral condyle
Medial tibial condyle	Medial femoral condyle	Tibial tuberosity
Fibular head ligament	Transverse ligament	Posterior cruciate
Anterior cruciate ligament		

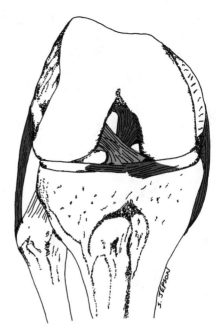

FIGURE 19-5 The right knee in flexion, anterior view.

8. On Figure 19-6, (a) draw in the origin and insertion of the muscles, and (b) join the origin and insertion to show the line of pull.

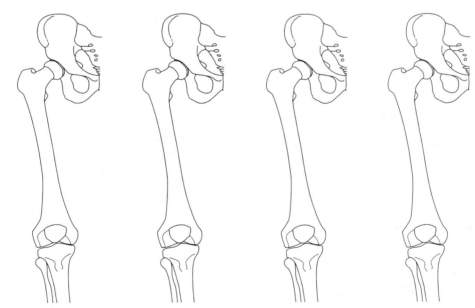

FIGURE 19-6 Rectus femoris, vastus medialis, vastus lateralis, vastus intermedialis.

9. On Figure 19-7, label the origin and insertion of the popliteus and gastrocnemius, joining the origin and insertion to show the line of pull.

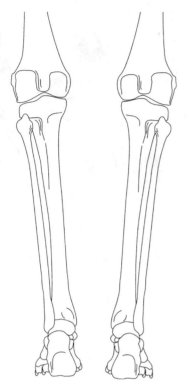

FIGURE 19-7 Popliteus and gastrocnemius.

10. Review semimembranosus, semitendinosus, and biceps femoris in Chapter 18.

11. For the knee joint, give the following information:

Joint	Shape	Degrees of Freedom	Motions	Plane	Axis
Knee					

12. At the knee joint, identify which surface is concave and which is convex.

Joint	Concave	Convex
Knee		

13. For the knee joint, provide the close-packed position and the loose-packed position (refer to Chapter 4, Table 4-4 for descriptions).

Joint	Close-Packed	Loose-Packed
Knee		

14. For the knee joint, describe the normal end feel (refer to Chapter 4, Table 4-1 for descriptions).

Flexion: _____ Bony _____ Soft tissue stretch
_____ Soft tissue approximation
Extension: _____ Bony _____ Soft tissue stretch
_____ Soft tissue approximation

15. Match each ligament and structure listed below with its appropriate function or characteristic. An answer may be used more than once. Each function or characteristic may have more than one correct answer.

_____ Posterior cruciate ligament

_____ Anterior cruciate ligament

_____ Lateral collateral ligament

_____ Medial collateral ligament

_____ Lateral meniscus

_____ Medial meniscus

A. Provides stability in the frontal plane

B. Prevents anterior displacement of the tibia on the femur

C. Fibers of the meniscus attach to this ligament

D. Deepens the joint surface

E. Prevents posterior displacement of the tibia on the femur

F. Absorbs shock

16. For each muscle listed, check the motions for which the muscle is a major contributor at the knee.

Muscle	Flexion	Extension
Vastus lateralis		
Vastus medialis		
Vastus intermedialis		
Rectus femoris		
Semimembranosus		
Semitendinosus		
Biceps femoris		
Popliteus		
Gastrocnemius		

17. Indicate the positions that simultaneously lengthen or shorten the multijoint muscles over all the joints they cross.

Muscle	Lengthened Position			Shortened Position		
	Hip	*Knee*	*Ankle*	*Hip*	*Knee*	*Ankle*
Rectus femoris						
Semimembranosus						
Semitendinosus						
Biceps femoris long head						
Gastrocnemius						

18. The sciatic nerve comes off of which nerve roots?

   _____

   On which side of the thigh is the sciatic nerve located?

   _____ Anterior _____ Posterior _____ Medial

   _____ Lateral

   List the two nerves that the sciatic nerve divides into at the knee.

   _____

   _____

19. Describe the general pathway of the two divisions of the sciatic nerve as they descend from the knee to the foot.

   _____

   _____

   _____

20. Describe the general pathway of the femoral nerve and then identify the knee muscles it innervates.

   _____

   _____

   _____

21. During terminal knee extension:

   A. In a closed kinetic chain, the femur rotates on the tibia in which direction?

   _____

   B. In an open kinetic chain, the tibia rotates on the femur in which direction?

   _____

22. What artery passes posterior to the knee?

   _____

■ ■ ■ Lab Activities

Student's Name _____

Date Due _____

1. Palpation of bones and landmarks, ligaments, and other structures:
   - Locate on bones and skeleton, and palpate when possible.
   - The reference position is the anatomical position.
   - Not all structures can be palpated on your partner.

Tibia

Intercondylar eminence	A double-pointed prominence centered on the proximal surface of the tibia. It extends into the intercondyloid fossa of the femur. Cannot be palpated.
Medial condyle	The proximal medial aspect of the tibia. Palpate below the joint space on the medial surface. **FIGURE 19-8** Palpating the medial condyle.
Lateral condyle	The proximal lateral aspect of the tibia. Palpate below the joint space on the lateral surface. **FIGURE 19-9** Palpating the lateral condyle.
Tibial plateau	The broad proximal end of the tibia, including the medial and lateral condyles and the intercondylar eminence

Tibial tuberosity	A protuberance on the proximal anterior midline of the tibia; the attachment for the patellar tendon. Palpate the patella and move your fingers distal to the insertion of the patellar tendon on the tibial tuberosity. See Figure 18-15.
Crest	The sharp anterior border along the ridge of the tibia. Palpate by moving your fingers distally from the tibial tuberosity along the crest. The crest is very superficial along most of its length.
Medial malleolus	Enlarged distal medial surface of the tibia. Palpate on the medial surface of the ankle. **FIGURE 19-10** Palpating the medial malleolus.

Fibula

Head	Enlarged proximal end of the fibula. Palpate on the lateral aspect of the knee. **FIGURE 19-11** Palpating the head of the fibula.

Continued

Fibula—Cont'd

Lateral malleolus	Enlarged distal lateral surface of the fibula. Palpate on the lateral aspect of the ankle. Note that the lateral malleolus extends further distally than the medial malleolus. **FIGURE 19-12** Palpating the lateral malleolus.

Other Structures

Patella	A triangular sesamoid bone on the anterior aspect of the knee. Palpate it on the anterior of the knee joint. With the person relaxed, move the patella in all directions, making note of the amount of ROM. When the knee is flexed, this movement is not possible. **FIGURE 19-13** Palpating the patella.
Posterior cruciate ligament	Located deep in the knee; attaches to the tibia posteriorly in the intercondylar area and runs in a superior and anterior direction to attach anteriorly on the medial condyle of the femur. It cannot be palpated.
Anterior cruciate ligament	Located deep in the knee; attaches to the tibia anteriorly in the intercondylar area and runs in a superior and posterior direction to attach posteriorly on the lateral condyle of the femur. It cannot be palpated.

Lateral collateral ligament	A cordlike structure located on the lateral aspect of the knee; attaches to the lateral condyle of the femur and the head of the fibula. With the knee in extension, palpate on the lateral surface of the knee by moving your fingers perpendicular to the weight-bearing surface of the tibia.
Medial collateral ligament	A flat, broad ligament on the medial surface; attaches to the medial condyle of the femur and to the medial tibial condyle. Fibers of the medial meniscus attach to this ligament. Palpate it on the medial aspect of the knee.
Lateral meniscus	Located deep within the knee on the weight-bearing surface of the lateral tibial condyle. It cannot be palpated.
Medial meniscus	Located deep within the knee on the weight-bearing surface of the medial tibial condyle. It cannot be palpated.
Calcaneus	Located on the posterior foot **FIGURE 19-14** Palpating the calcaneus.

2. Palpation of muscles:

A. Locate the following muscles on the skeleton and anatomical models, and on at least one partner.

- The information needed to palpate each muscle is provided.
- The position described for locating the muscle on your partner is usually the manual muscle test position for a fair or better grade of muscle strength.
- Not all origins, insertions, and muscle bellies can be palpated on your partner.

B. On the skeleton, locate the origin and insertion of each muscle.

- Place the ends of a rubber band at the origin and insertion of the muscle, making the band taut. Note the location of the muscle in relation to the joints it crosses.

- When possible, move the skeleton to perform the motion of the muscle, observing how the rubber band becomes less taut, similar to the change in length of the muscle as the muscle performs a concentric contraction.

- Return the skeleton to the starting position and observe how the rubber band becomes taut, similar to the change in length of the muscle as the muscle performs an eccentric contraction.

C. When possible, locate each muscle on your partner and palpate the origin, insertion, and muscle belly of each muscle. Asking your partner to contract and relax the muscle while you palpate ensures that you are on the correct muscle.

Sitting Position

RECTUS FEMORIS:	Superficial on the anterior thigh. See Figure 18-18.
Position of person:	With hip and knee flexed
Origin:	Anterior inferior iliac spine
Insertion:	Tibial tuberosity via the patellar tendon
Line of pull:	Vertical on the anterior surface of the thigh and over the knee joint
Muscle action:	Knee extension, hip flexion
Palpate:	Palpate along the midline of the thigh or at the patellar tendon. The origin can be isolated by palpating the tendon as it crosses the hip joint.
Instructions to person:	Straighten your knee.

VASTUS LATERALIS:	Superficial on the anterior lateral thigh
	FIGURE 19-15 Palpating the right vastus lateralis.
Position of person:	With hip and knee flexed
Origin:	Linea aspera
Insertion:	Tibial tuberosity via the patellar tendon
Line of pull:	Vertical on the anterior surface of the thigh and over the knee joint
Muscle action:	Knee extension
Palpate:	Palpate on the lateral portion of the thigh or at the patellar tendon
Instructions to person:	Straighten your knee.
VASTUS MEDIALIS:	Superficial on the anterior medial thigh
	FIGURE 19-16 Palpating the right vastus medialis.
Position of person:	With hip and knee flexed

Continued

Sitting Position—Cont'd

Origin:	Linea aspera of the femur
Insertion:	Tibial tuberosity via the patellar tendon
Line of pull:	Vertical on the anterior surface of the thigh and over the knee joint
Muscle action:	Knee extension
Palpate:	Palpate along the medial portion of the thigh or the patellar tendon
Instructions to person:	Straighten your knee.
VASTUS INTERMEDIALIS:	Deep to the rectus femoris on the anterior thigh
Position of person:	Hip and knee flexed
Origin:	Anterior femur
Insertion:	Tibial tuberosity via the patellar tendon
Line of pull:	Vertical on the anterior surface of the thigh and over the knee joint
Muscle action:	Knee extension
Palpate:	Cannot palpate directly because it is deep to the rectus femoris and does not have a separate action.
Instructions to person:	Straighten your knee.

Prone Position

SEMITENDINOSUS:	A superficial muscle on the posterior medial aspect of the thigh. See Figure 18-22.
Position of person:	Hip extended and knee flexed, and in neutral alignment
Origin:	Ischial tuberosity
Insertion:	Proximal anterior medial tibia
Line of pull:	Vertical on the posterior surface of the thigh and the hip and knee joints
Muscle action:	Hip extension and knee flexion

Palpate:	Palpate on the posterior medial thigh. The long distal tendon is on the distal medial aspect of the thigh, superficial to the attachment of the semimembranosus.
Instructions to person:	Keep your knee bent and don't let me straighten it.
SEMIMEMBRANOSUS:	Deep to the semitendinosus muscle and located on the posterior medial thigh. See Figure 18-23.
Position of person:	Hip extended and knee flexed, and in neutral alignment
Origin:	Ischial tuberosity
Insertion:	Posterior surface of the medial condyle of the tibia
Line of pull:	Vertical on the posterior surface of the thigh and the hip and knee joints
Muscle action:	Hip extension and knee flexion
Palpate:	Palpate on the posterior medial thigh. Distinguishing between the semimembranosus and the semitendinosus can be difficult. The semimembranosus has a broad attachment on the posterior surface of the tibia deep to and on either side of the semitendinosus, just above the knee joint.
Instructions to person:	Keep your knee bent and don't let me straighten it.
BICEPS FEMORIS:	A superficial muscle on the posterior lateral thigh. See Figure 18-24.
Position of person:	Hip extended and knee flexed, and in neutral alignment
Origin:	Long head: Ischial tuberosity Short head: Lateral lip of the linea aspera of the femur
Insertion:	Posterior proximal fibular head
Line of pull:	Vertical on the posterior surface of the thigh and the hip and knee joints

Muscle action:	Long head: Hip extension and knee flexion Short head: Knee flexion
Palpate:	On the posterior lateral thigh. The tendon is palpated on the distal lateral thigh at the knee joint.
Instructions to person:	Keep your knee bent and don't let me straighten it.
POPLITEUS:	Deep to the gastrocnemius on the posterior proximal leg
Position of person:	Hip and knee extended in neutral alignment
Origin:	Lateral condyle of the femur
Insertion:	Posterior medial condyle of the tibia
Line of pull:	Diagonal on the posterior surface of the knee joint
Muscle action:	Initiates knee flexion
Palpate:	Cannot be palpated
Instructions to person:	Flex your knee.

Standing Position

GASTROCNEMIUS:	Superficial on the posterior of the leg
	FIGURE 19-17 Palpating the gastrocnemius.
Position of person:	Hip and knee extended, ankle in neutral
Origin:	Posterior aspect of the medial and lateral condyles of the femur

Insertion:	Via a common tendon onto the posterior aspect of the calcaneus
Line of pull:	Vertical
Muscle action:	Ankle plantar flexion
Palpate:	Palpate on the posterior proximal medial and lateral aspects of the leg
Instructions to person:	Rise up on your toes.

3. Observe the amount of motion available at the knee joint in the sagittal plane and estimate the degrees of flexion by checking the box that *most closely* describes that amount of motion. (Do not measure with a goniometer.)

Motions	0°–45°	46°–90°	91°–135°	136°–180°
Flexion				

4. Passively move your partner through the available range of motion, making note of the end feel. If possible, repeat with several people. Review worksheet question 12 about normal end feel.

   A. Is your partner's end feel consistent with normal end feel? _____

   B. What structures create the end feel for this joint?

   _____

   _____

5. Using a disarticulated skeleton or anatomical model of the knee joint, apply the rules of joint arthrokinematics and the concave-convex rule to perform the following exercises.

   A. Underline the correct answer.

   The femur is concave/convex.

   The tibia is concave/convex.

   B. Move the tibia on the femur in all planes of motion.

   C. Observe the movement of the tibia on the femur. Circle the motions that you observed.

   Roll   Spin   Glide

6. Referring to pre-lab worksheet 17, assume the positions that make the multijoint muscles:

   A. Lengthen simultaneously over all the joints they cross.

   Hamstrings: _____

   Quadriceps: _____

   B. This can result in which type of insufficiency?

   _____

   C. Shorten simultaneously over all the joints they cross.

   Hamstrings: _____

   Quadriceps: _____

   D. This can result in which type of insufficiency?

   _____

7. With your partner standing, observe from the front to determine whether genu valgus and genu varus is present. Does your partner have

   genu valgus _____ genu varus _____
   normal alignment _____

8. With your partner supine, measure the Q angle using a goniometer. Place the axis of the goniometer over the midpoint of the patella. Align one arm of the goniometer with the AIIS and the other arm with the tibial tuberosity.

   A. How does your partner's Q angle compare to normal range of the Q angle?

   _____

   B. Do the angles of the right and left lower extremities appear equal?

   _____

9. The knee generally has a few degrees of motion in the sagittal plane beyond 0° of extension.

   A. What is this motion called? _____

   B. What structures allow this motion? _____

   C. What term is used to describe an excessive amount of this motion?

   _____

D. Starting in the long sitting position, ask your partner to extend the knee as much as possible. Normally, the heel will rise less than an inch. Does your partner's heel come off the table, and if so by how many inches?

_____

E. With your partner standing, observe from the side and describe your partner's knee position.

_____

10. **Functional activity analysis:**

    In each chapter on the lower extremity, you will be analyzing the activity of moving from sitting to standing, and the reverse motion of moving from standing to sitting. Perform these activities and then analyze how the subject in Figures 19-18 through 19-22 performed those activities.

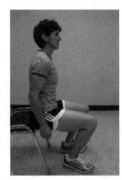

FIGURE 19-18 Starting position to assume standing.

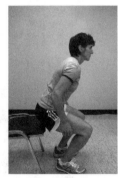

FIGURE 19-19 Initiating standing.

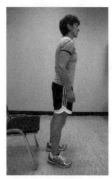

FIGURE 19-20 Ending position for standing. Starting position for sitting down.

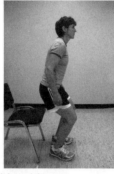

FIGURE 19-21 Midposition.

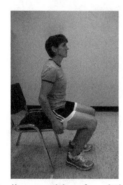

FIGURE 19-22 Ending position for sitting.

A. Describe the positions of the knee when the subject is:

1) moving from sitting to standing. _____

_____

2) moving from standing to sitting. _____

_____

B. Which muscle groups are acting as prime movers in the following motions?

1) Moving from sitting to standing _____

_____

2) Moving from standing to sitting _____

_____

C. Describe the type of muscle contraction being used, when, and why:

1) moving from sitting to standing. _____

_____

2) moving from standing to sitting. _____

_____

D. Explain your answers to part C.

1) Moving from sitting to standing _____

_____

2) Moving from standing to sitting _____

_____

11. Using washable markers, draw on your partner the paths of the:

A. Femoral nerve

B. Sciatic nerve, including the branching of the tibial and common peroneal nerves (need not go beyond proximal end of leg).

C. Femoral artery and vein.

D. Popliteal artery, showing branching of anterior and posterior tibial arteries.

E. Popliteal vein, showing connection with small saphenous vein.

F. Great saphenous vein, showing connection with femoral vein.

■ ■ ■ Post-Lab Questions

Student's Name _____

Date Due _____

After you have completed the worksheets and lab activities, answer the following questions without using your book or notes. When finished, check your answers.

1. In considering various impairments of the knee, you are reviewing the muscles that attach distal to the knee and proximal to the pelvis. Starting anteriorly and moving medially around the knee, name the multijoint muscles that cross the hip and knee.

   _____

   _____

2. In considering various impairments of the ankle, you are reviewing the muscles that attach proximal on the femur and distally on the calcaneus. List the multijoint muscle(s) that cross the knee and attach posteriorly on the calcaneus.

   _____

3. Which muscle of the hamstrings group does not cross the hip?

   _____

4. Which muscle of the quadriceps muscle group crosses the hip? _____

5. Starting at the tibial tuberosity and proceeding laterally around the knee, name, in order, the muscles that span the knee joint.

   _____

   _____

6. Describe the positions that make the hamstrings group actively insufficient.

   Hip _____ Knee _____

   Describe the positions that make the hamstrings group passively insufficient.

   Hip _____ Knee _____

7. Describe the positions that make the rectus femoris actively insufficient.

   Hip _____ Knee _____

   Describe the positions that make the rectus femoris passively insufficient.

   Hip _____ Knee _____

8. Why is the Q angle of women generally larger than the Q angle of men?

   _____

9. Identify the varus and valgus changes at the hips and knees in Figures 19-23 and 19-24.

   A. Coxa _____ B. Genu _____

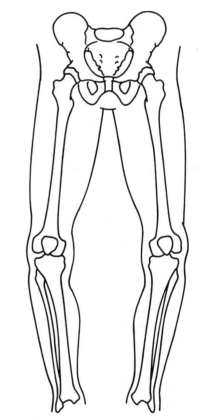

FIGURE 19-23 Hip and knee varus and valgus.

A. Coxa _____ B. Genu _____

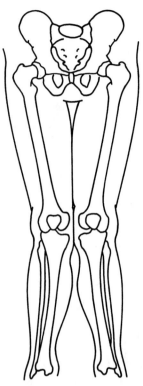

FIGURE 19-24 Hip and knee varus and valgus.

10. Name the muscles that make up the pes anserine muscle group.

_____

11. A. What knee flexor is innervated by the common peroneal nerve?

_____

   B. Is it located on the _____ medial or _____ lateral side of the posterior knee?

12. A. The popliteus muscle has its proximal attachment on which side of the posterior knee?

   ` _____ Medial _____ Lateral

   B. The popliteus muscle is innervated by which nerve? _____

13. Indicate the location of the following bursae:

Bursae	Location
Subcutaneous infrapatellar	
Deep infrapatellar	
Gastrocnemius	
Fibular collateral ligament	

14. The popliteal fossa has many vital structures passing through it.

   A. The muscle(s) that make up the superior medial border are the _____.

   B. The muscle(s) that make up the superior lateral border are the _____.

   C. The muscle(s) that make up the inferior medial and lateral borders are the _____.

   D. The nerve that passes through the middle of the fossa is the _____.

   E. The nerve that passes through the fossa on the lateral border is the _____.

   F. The artery and vein that pass through the fossa are the _____.

   G. The vein that enters the fossa inferiorly to join the vein is the _____.

   H. The muscle that forms the floor is the

   _____.

15. The femoral condyles act as simple pulleys for the tendons of which three muscles?

   _____

16. What might be some of the effects on the weight-bearing surfaces of the knee when the line of gravity does not fall in the normal position through the knee joint because of varus, valgus, or recurvatum?

   _____

   _____

Ankle Joint and Foot

■ ■ ■ Pre-Lab Worksheets

Student's Name _____

Date Due _____

Complete the following questions prior to the lab class.

1. Match the following terms with the appropriate descriptions.

_____ Equinus   A. Abnormally high arch

_____ Pes cavus   B. Valgus deformity of great toe

_____ Pes planus   C. Hindfoot fixed in plantar flexion

_____ Hallux valgus   D. Abnormally low arch

2. Match the parts of the foot with the bones that make up that part.

_____ Hindfoot   A. Five metatarsals and all the phalanges

_____ Midfoot   B. Talus and calcaneus

_____ Forefoot   C. Navicular, cuboid, and three cuneiforms

3. On Figure 20-1:

A. Identify the view.

A. _____ B. _____ C. _____

B. Label the following bones and landmarks:

Tarsals: Talus   Cuboid

Calcaneus: Sustentaculum tali

Cuneiforms: 1–3

Navicular: Tuberosity of the navicular

Metatarsals: Base   Head

Phalanges:

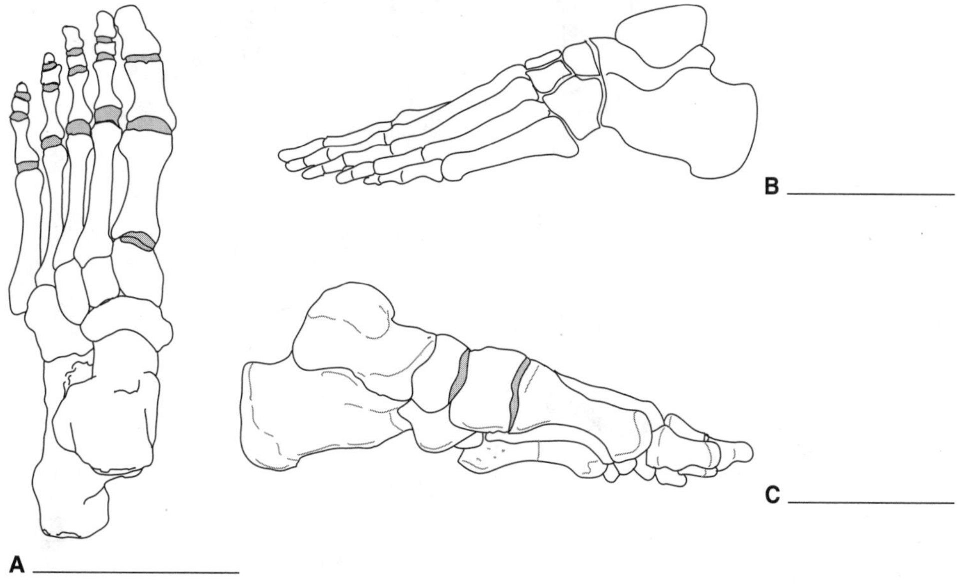

A _____

B _____

C _____

FIGURE 20-1 Views, bones, and landmarks of the foot.

4. On Figure 20-2, label the bones, landmarks, and
   ligaments.

BONES: Tibia   Fibula
LANDMARKS: Crest   Medial malleolus
                    Head   Lateral malleolus
LIGAMENTS: Superior   Inferior
                        tibiofibular   tibiofibular
                    Interosseous membrane

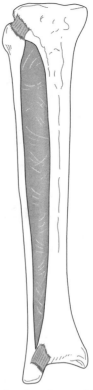

FIGURE 20-2 Bones, landmarks, and ligaments of the leg.

5. A. On Figure 20-3, label the joints and identify the bones that make up the joints of the ankle.

JOINTS: Talocrural   Subtalar   Transverse tarsal
BONES: Tibia   Talus   Fibula
          Calcaneus   Navicular   Cuboid

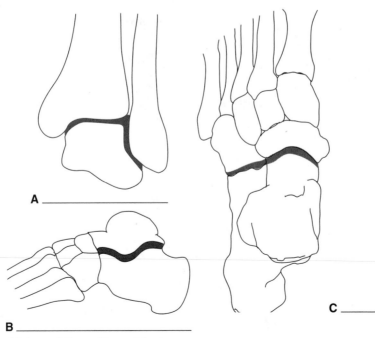

A _____

B _____

C _____

FIGURE 20-3 Bones and joints of the ankle and foot.

B. On Figure 20-4, label the joints and bones that make up the forefoot.

Metatarsophalangeal (MTP), tarsometatarsal

Interphalangeal: proximal (PIP), distal (DIP), and interphalangeal (IP)

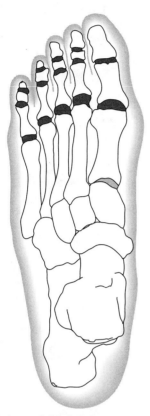

FIGURE 20-4 Joints of the forefoot.

6. Label the bones and ligaments on Figures 20-5 through 20-7.

BONES: Cuboid Metatarsals Tibia Navicular
Talus Calcaneus Cuneiforms Fibula

LIGAMENTS:

A. Label the four parts of the deltoid ligament:

Posterior tibiotalar ligament   Anterior tibiotalar ligament

Tibionavicular ligament   Tibiocalcaneal ligament

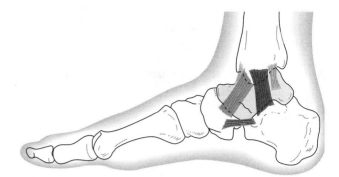

FIGURE 20-5 Bones and ligaments of the right medial ankle.

B. Label the three parts of the lateral ligament:

Posterior talofibular ligament   Anterior talofibular ligament

Calcaneofibular ligament

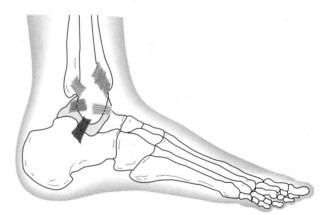

FIGURE 20-6 Bones and ligaments of the right lateral ankle.

C.

Spring ligament   Long plantar ligament

Short plantar ligament   Plantar aponeurosis

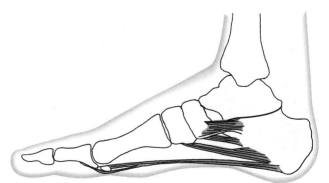

FIGURE 20-7 Bones and ligaments of the right medial foot.

7. On Figures 20-8A, B, and C, label the arches and the bones making up those arches.

ARCHES: Medial longitudinal   Lateral longitudinal
                    arch   arch
            Transverse arch

A. _____ B. _____ C. _____

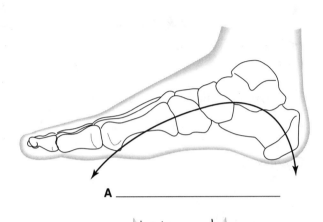 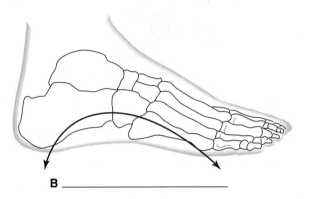

A _____

B _____

C _____

FIGURE 20-8 Arches of the foot.

8. On Figures 20-9 through 20-16:

   A. Label the origin and insertion of the muscles shown.

   B. Join the origin and insertion to show the line of pull.

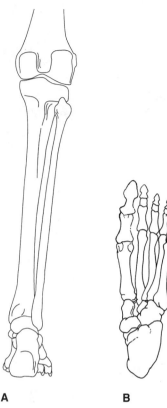

A   **B**

FIGURE 20-11 **(A)** and **(B)** Flexor hallucis longus.

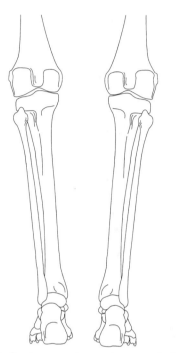

FIGURE 20-9 Gastrocnemius, soleus, and plantaris.

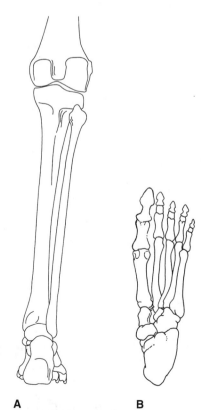

A   **B**

FIGURE 20-10 **(A)** and **(B)** Tibialis posterior.

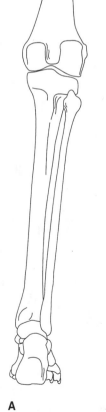
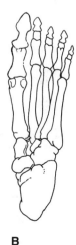

A   **B**

FIGURE 20-12 **(A)** and **(B)** Flexor digitorum longus.

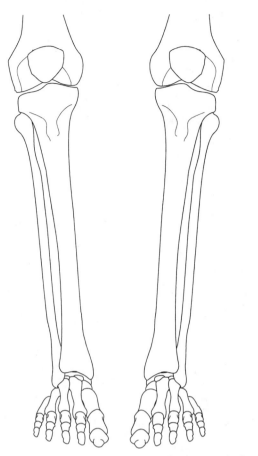

FIGURE 20-13 Tibialis anterior and extensor hallucis longus.

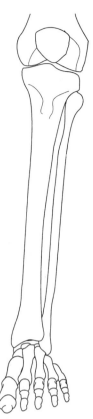

FIGURE 20-14 Extensor digitorum longus.

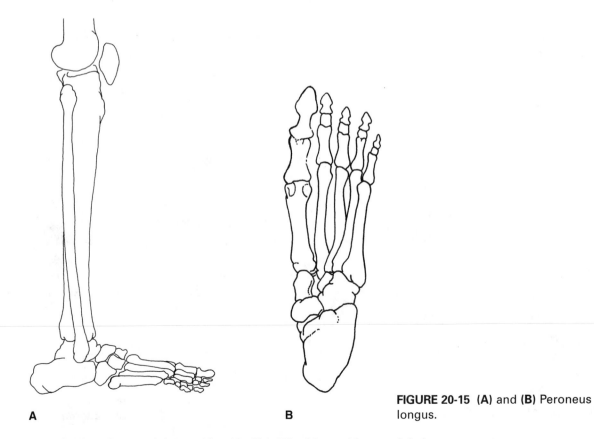

A   B

FIGURE 20-15 **(A)** and **(B)** Peroneus longus.

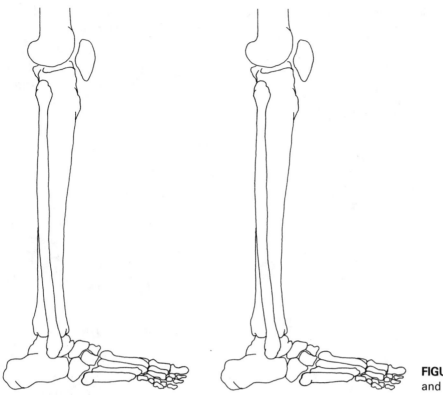

FIGURE 20-16 Peroneus brevis and peroneus tertius.

9. For each of the joints listed, give the following information:

Joint	Shape	Degrees of Freedom	Motions
Talocrural			
Metatarsophalangeal			
Interphalangeal of great toe			

10. A. At each of the following joints, identify which surface is concave and which is convex.

Joint	Concave	Convex
Talocrural		
Metatarsophalangeal		
Interphalangeal of great toe		

B. Describe the arthrokinematics when performing flexion of the MTP joint of the great toe.

_____

11. For each of the following joints, provide the close-packed position and the loose-packed position (refer to Chapter 4, Table 4-4 for descriptions).

Joint	Close-Packed	Loose-Packed
Talocrural		
Subtalar		
Transverse tarsal		

12. For each of the following joints, describe the normal end feel (refer to Chapter 4, Table 4-1 for descriptions).

Joints	Bony	Soft Tissue Stretch	Soft Tissue Approximation
Talocrural			
Subtalar			
Metatarso-phalangeal of great toe			

13. Match each ligament and structure listed below with the appropriate function or characteristic. Use each answer once.

_____ Deltoid ligament

_____ Medial longitudinal arch

_____ Spring ligament

_____ Plantar aponeurosis

_____ Transverse arch

_____ Lateral ligament

A. Three parts, each with an insertion on the fibula

B. Located on the medial side, triangular in shape

C. Runs from side to side at the distal row of tarsals

D. Supports the medial side of the longitudinal arch

E. The talus is the keystone

F. Supports both longitudinal arches

14. For each muscle listed, check the motions for which it is a prime mover.

Muscle	Plantar Flexion	Dorsiflexion	Eversion	Inversion	Flexion	Extension
Gastrocnemius						
Soleus						
Plantaris*						
Tibialis posterior						
Flexor hallucis longus						
Flexor digitorum longus						
Tibialis anterior						
Extensor hallucis longus						
Extensor digitorum longus						
Peroneus longus						
Peroneus brevis						
Peroneus tertius*						

* Muscle's only role is as an assistive mover.

15. For the multijoint muscles listed, indicate the joints they cross, and the positions that simultaneously lengthen or shorten them over all the joints they cross.

Muscle	Lengthened Position				Shortened Position			
	Knee	Ankle	Foot	MP, IP	Knee	Ankle	Foot	MP, IP
Gastrocnemius								
Soleus								
Plantaris								
Tibialis posterior								
Flexor hallucis longus								
Flexor digitorum longus								
Tibialis anterior								
Extensor hallucis longus								
Extensor digitorum								
Peroneus longus								
Peroneus brevis								
Peroneus tertius								

16. Place your left hand on the medial side of your right ankle with your index, middle, and ring fingers just posterior to the medial malleolus. Name the artery and nerve located approximately between your middle and ring fingers. _____

■ ■ ■ Lab Activities

Student's Name _____

Date Due _____

1. Palpation of bones and landmarks, ligaments, and other structures:
   - Locate on bones and skeleton, and palpate when possible.
   - The reference position is the anatomical position.
   - Not all structures can be palpated on your partner.

Tarsal Bones and Landmarks

Calcaneus	The largest and most posterior tarsal bone; also called the heel. Palpate by grasping the heel. See Figure 19-14.
Calcaneal tuberosity	The rounded area on the posterior surface
Sustentaculum tali	A small protuberance on the proximal medial side of the calcaneus. Palpate the medial malleolus, and then move your finger distal about two finger-widths. The tip may be more distinct with the ankle passively inverted.
Talus	Located between the tibia and calcaneus. With the foot in plantar flexion, the talus can be palpated on the dorsum of the foot distal to the tibia. The talus can also be palpated between the navicular tuberosity and the medial malleolus.

FIGURE 20-17 Palpating the talus.

Navicular	Located on the medial side of the foot between the talus and the cuneiforms. Palpate on the dorsum and medial side of the foot.
Tuberosity of the navicular	A protuberance on the medial surface of the navicular. Palpate on the medial side of the foot distal to the medial malleolus. Palpation is easier with the foot inverted because the tuberosity becomes more pronounced.

FIGURE 20-18 Palpating the navicular tuberosity.

Cuboid	Located on the lateral side of the foot between the calcaneus and the metatarsals. Palpate its flat surface on the lateral side of the foot. Place one finger on the base of the fifth metatarsal and one finger on the lateral malleolus. The cuboid is located between the two fingers just proximal to the fifth metatarsal.

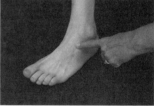

FIGURE 20-19 Palpating the cuboid.

Continued

Tarsal Bones and Landmarks—Cont'd

Cuneiforms: 1–3	The first cuneiform is located on the medial side of the foot, the second is lateral to the first, and the third is between the second and the cuboid. The cuneiforms are between the navicular and the metatarsals. Palpate starting from the medial side of the foot and moving laterally. Locate the first metatarsal and slide your finger proximal to the indentation of the first TMT joint. The first cuneiform is just proximal. Move your finger laterally along the dorsal surface to the second and third cuneiforms. 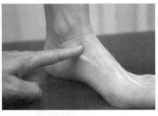 **FIGURE 20-20** Palpating the cuneiforms.

Metatarsals

First–fifth	Located between the tarsals (cuneiforms and cuboid) and the phalanges. Palpate between the tarsals and the phalanges from medial to lateral. 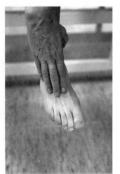 **FIGURE 20-21** Palpating the metatarsals.
Base	Proximal end of each metatarsal
Head	Distal end of each metatarsal
First	Thickest and shortest, located on medial side of the foot. It articulates with the great toe.

Second	The longest; articulates with the second cuneiform and the second toe.
Third	Articulates with the third cuneiform and the third toe
Fourth	Articulates with the cuboid and the fourth toe
Fifth	Articulates with the cuboid and the fifth toe

Phalanges

Great toe (first)	Two—proximal, distal
Lesser toes (second–fifth)	Three each—proximal, middle, distal

Joints

Superior tibiofibular	Articulation between the head of the fibula and the proximal posterior lateral aspect of the tibia. Palpate just above the fibular head.
Inferior tibiofibular	Articulation between the distal tibia and the distal fibula on the lateral side of the ankle. Palpate an indentation just medial to the anterior edge of the lateral malleolus.
Talocrural or talotibial or ankle	Articulation between the tibia and talus. First, palpate the distal tip of the medial and lateral malleoli. Next, move the finger from the medial malleolus (tibia) to a finger's width distal to palpate the talus.
Subtalar or talocalcaneal	Articulation of the inferior surface of the talus with the superior surface of the calcaneus. Difficult to palpate.
Transverse tarsal or midtarsal	Articulations of the anterior surface of the talus and calcaneus with the navicular and cuboid, respectively. Palpate slightly anterior between the navicular tuberosity and the medial malleolus, and between the cuboid and lateral malleolus.

Tarsometatarsal	Articulations of the cuneiforms and cuboid with the metatarsals.
Metatarsophalangeal	Articulations between the respective metatarsals and proximal phalanges of the toes.
Interphalangeal	Articulations between the proximal and distal phalanges of the great toe and between the proximal and middle and middle and distal phalanges of the lesser toes.

Ligaments and Other Structures

Joint capsule	Surrounds the ankle joint and is reinforced by ligaments. Cannot be palpated.
Deltoid ligament: tibionavicular, tibiocalcaneal, posterior tibiotalar, and anterior tibiotalar	Triangular ligament on the medial side of the ankle joint; attachments are a narrow proximal attachment on the tip of the medial malleolus and broader distal attachment on the talus, navicular, and calcaneus. Palpate on the medial side of the foot just distal to the medial malleolus. Move your finger anterior and posterior as the foot is moved in eversion and inversion.
Lateral ligament: anterior talofibular, posterior talofibular, and calcaneofibular	On lateral side of the ankle joining the lateral malleolus to the talus and calcaneus. The weak anterior talofibular ligament attaches the lateral malleolus to the talus anteriorly. The stronger posterior talofibular ligament is horizontal, connecting the lateral malleolus to the talus posteriorly. The calcaneofibular ligament is located between the anterior and posterior talofibular ligaments and is a long, fairly vertical ligament joining the lateral malleolus to the calcaneus. Palpate on the lateral side of the foot distal to the lateral malleolus to feel the calcaneofibular ligament. Move your fingers anteriorly and posteriorly as the foot is moved in inversion and eversion to feel the anterior and posterior talofibular ligaments, respectively.
Medial longitudinal arch	A proximal-distal arch on the medial border of the foot consisting of the calcaneus, talus, navicular, three cuneiforms, and the first three metatarsals. Observe the medial border of the foot both in weight-bearing and non-weight-bearing.
Lateral longitudinal arch	A proximal-distal arch on the lateral border of the foot consisting of the calcaneus, cuboid, and third and fourth metatarsals. Observe the lateral border of the foot. Note that there appears to be very little visible arch.
Transverse arch	A side-to-side arch in the midfoot consisting of the three cuneiforms and the cuboid. To accentuate the arch, press up in the middle of the plantar surface of the foot over the heads of the metatarsals. A callus in this area tends to be indicative of a low transverse arch.
Spring ligament or plantar calcaneonavicular	A short, wide ligament on the medial side supporting the medial longitudinal arch. Attaches from the calcaneus to the navicular. Palpate deeply just posterior to the navicular tuberosity. Roll your finger vertically over the ligament.
Long plantar ligament	Superficial. Attaches to the calcaneus and runs forward to attach on the cuboid and bases of the third, fourth, and fifth metatarsals. Supports the lateral longitudinal arch. Difficult to separate from the short plantar ligament when palpating.
Short plantar ligament	Deep to the long plantar ligament on the lateral side of the foot; it attaches to the calcaneus and cuboid. Difficult to separate from long plantar ligament when palpating.
Plantar aponeurosis	Superficial on the plantar surface of the foot. It supports both longitudinal arches; attaches to the calcaneus and the proximal phalanges. Palpate on the plantar surface anterior to the calcaneus while hyperextending the toes.

2. Palpation of muscles:

A. Locate the following muscles on the skeleton and anatomical models, and on at least one partner.

- The information needed to palpate each muscle is provided in the following tables.
- For a fair or better grade of muscle strength, the position described for locating the muscle on your partner is usually the manual muscle test position.
- Not all origins, insertions, and muscle bellies can be palpated on your partner.

B. On the skeleton, locate the origin and insertion of each muscle.

- Place the ends of a rubber band at the origin and insertion of the muscle, making the band taut. Note the location of the muscle in relation to the joints it crosses.
- When possible, move the skeleton to perform the muscle's motion and observe how the band becomes less taut, similar to the change in length as it performs a concentric contraction.

Standing Position

GASTROCNEMIUS:	Located superficially on the posterior leg. See Figure 19-17.
Position of person:	With ankle in neutral or with a few degrees of dorsiflexion and the knee in extension
Origin:	Medial head: Posterior on medial condyle of femur Lateral head: Posterior on lateral condyle of femur
Insertion:	Posterior calcaneus
Line of pull:	Vertical
Muscle action:	Ankle plantar flexion, knee flexion
Palpate:	Posterior aspect of the leg in the upper-third region
Instructions to person:	Rise up on your toes.

SOLEUS:	Located deep to the gastrocnemius on the posterior leg

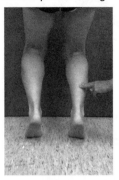

FIGURE 20-22 Palpating the soleus.

Position of person:	With ankle in neutral or a few degrees of dorsiflexion and the knee in partial flexion
Origin:	Posterior tibia and fibula
Insertion:	Posterior calcaneus
Line of pull:	Vertical
Muscle action:	Ankle plantar flexion
Palpate:	Distal to, and on both sides of, the muscle belly of the gastrocnemius
Instructions to person:	Keeping your knee slightly bent, rise up on your toes.
PLANTARIS:	Located deep to the lateral head of the gastrocnemius
Position of person:	With ankle in neutral and the knee flexed
Origin:	Posterior lateral condyle of the femur
Insertion:	Posterior calcaneus
Line of pull:	Vertical on the posterior side of the lower leg and ankle
Muscle action:	Assists in ankle plantar flexion

Palpate:	Locate the fibular head. Move your fingers medially into the popliteal space. Moving your fingers slightly proximal moves you away from the heads of the gastrocnemius. Press deeply. Difficult to palpate because it is very thin and doesn't have different action from gastrocnemius or soleus.
Instructions to person:	Point your toes.

Sitting Position

TIBIALIS POSTERIOR:	Muscle belly is deep to the soleus and gastrocnemius; tendon passes posterior to medial malleolus and around the medial side of the foot to its insertions.
	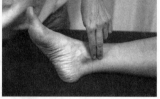 FIGURE 20-23 Palpating the tibialis posterior.
Position of person:	Sitting or supine, foot unsupported
Origin:	Interosseous membrane, adjacent tibia, and fibula
Insertion:	Navicular and most tarsals and metatarsals
Line of pull:	Vertical on the posterior surface of the lower leg and ankle
Muscle action:	Inversion; assists with plantar flexion
Palpate:	The tendon can be palpated behind the medial malleolus in the space between the malleolus and the Achilles tendon. The tendon can also be palpated between the medial malleolus and the navicular through it. It is

difficult to distinguish between the tendons of the tibialis posterior, flexor hallucis longus, and flexor digitorum longus. Palpating distal to the medial malleolus while moving the ankle and toes can assist in differentiating among these tendons.

Instructions to person:	Point your toes down and in.
FLEXOR HALLUCIS LONGUS:	Muscle belly is deep to the soleus and gastrocnemius; tendon passes posterior to the medial malleolus and around the medial side of the foot to its insertions.
	FIGURE 20-24 Palpating the flexor hallucis longus.
Position of person:	Foot supported in neutral
Origin:	Posterior fibula and interosseous membrane
Insertion:	Distal phalange of the great toe
Line of pull:	Vertical on the posterior surface of the lower leg and ankle
Muscle action:	Flexes the great toe at the MP and IP joints; assists inversion and plantar flexion of the ankle
Palpate:	The tendon is palpated posterior and inferior to the medial malleolus and on the medial side of the foot at the head of the great toe, distal to the medial malleolus (same as the tibialis posterior).

Continued

Sitting Position—Cont'd

Instructions to person:	Curl your toes.
FLEXOR DIGITORUM LONGUS:	Muscle belly is deep to the soleus and gastrocnemius; tendon passes posterior to the medial malleolus and around the medial side of the foot to its insertions.
Position of person:	With ankle in neutral
Origin:	Posterior tibia
Insertion:	Distal phalanges of the four lesser toes
Line of pull:	Vertical on the posterior surface of the lower leg and ankle
Muscle action:	Flexes the four lesser toes and assists in ankle inversion and plantar flexion
Palpate:	Posterior to the medial malleolus and along the medial aspect of the foot (same as tibialis posterior)
Instructions to person:	Curl your toes.
TIBIALIS ANTERIOR:	Located superficially on the anterior lateral leg

FIGURE 20-25 Palpating the tibialis anterior.

Position of person:	Ankle in neutral
Origin:	Lateral tibia and interosseous membrane
Insertion:	First cuneiform and metatarsal
Line of pull:	Vertical on the anterior surface of the lower leg and ankle

Muscle action:	Ankle inversion and dorsiflexion
Palpate:	Palpate the belly on the anterior lateral aspect of the tibia by identifying the tibial shaft and moving your fingers just lateral. Palpate the tendon as it crosses anteriorly to the medial side of the ankle.
Instructions to person:	Bring your foot up and in.
EXTENSOR HALLUCIS LONGUS:	Muscle belly is deep to the tibialis anterior and extensor digitorum longus muscles; tendon is on the dorsum of the foot. Tip of examiner's index finger is on tendon.

FIGURE 20-26 Palpating the extensor hallucis longus.

Position of person:	Ankle in neutral
Origin:	Anterior fibula and interosseous membrane
Insertion:	Distal phalange of the great toe
Line of pull:	Vertical on the anterior surface of the lower leg and ankle
Muscle action:	Extends the great toe; assists in ankle inversion and dorsiflexion
Palpate:	Palpate and observe the tendon as it crosses the ankle and on the dorsum of the foot leading to the insertion on the great toe
Instructions to person:	Straighten your great toe, pointing it to the ceiling.
EXTENSOR DIGITORUM LONGUS:	Muscle belly is deep to the tibialis anterior. See Figure 20-26. Tendons can be seen going to each of the four lesser toes.
Position of person:	Ankle in neutral

Origin:	Anterior fibula, interosseous membrane, and anterior lateral tibia
Insertion:	Dorsum of the distal phalanges of the four lesser toes
Line of pull:	Vertical on the anterior surface of the lower leg and ankle
Muscle action:	Extends four lesser toes, assists in ankle dorsiflexion
Palpate:	Palpate and observe the four tendons on the dorsum of the foot leading to the four lesser toes
Instructions to person:	Straighten your toes and point them to the ceiling.
PERONEUS LONGUS:	Located on the anterior lateral side of the leg, partially covered by the tibialis anterior and superficial to the other peroneal muscles

FIGURE 20-27 Palpating the peroneus longus.

Position of person:	Ankle and foot in neutral
Origin:	Proximal lateral fibula and interosseous membrane
Insertion:	Plantar surface of the first cuneiform and metatarsal
Line of pull:	Vertical on the lateral surface of the lower leg and ankle
Muscle action:	Ankle eversion; assists in plantar flexion
Palpate:	The muscle belly can be palpated on the lateral side distal to the head of the fibula and the lateral malleolus. The tendon is palpated posterior to the lateral malleolus before going deep on the plantar surface of the foot
Instructions to person:	Point your toes and move your foot to the outside.

PERONEUS BREVIS:	The muscle belly is deep to the peroneus longus on the distal lateral leg.
Position of person:	Ankle and foot in neutral
Origin:	Distal lateral fibula
Insertion:	Base of the fifth metatarsal
Line of pull:	Vertical on the lateral surface of the lower leg and ankle
Muscle action:	Ankle eversion; assists in plantar flexion.
Palpate:	The muscle belly is palpated on the distal lateral fibula but cannot be distinguished from the peroneus longus. The tendon can be palpated inferior to the lateral malleolus as it goes to its insertion on the base of the fifth metatarsal.
Instructions to person:	Move your foot to the outside.
PERONEUS TERTIUS:	The muscle belly is deep to the peroneus longus and the extensor digitorum longus on the distal anterior lateral leg.
Position of person:	Ankle and foot in neutral
Origin:	Distal medial fibula
Insertion:	Base of the fifth metatarsal
Line of pull:	Vertical on the lateral side of the ankle
Muscle action:	Assists in ankle eversion and dorsiflexion
Palpate:	The tendon is palpated from anterior to the lateral malleolus on the dorsum of the foot to the insertion on the head of the fifth metatarsal. It is not easily seen or palpated on all individuals. Do not confuse it with the tendon of the extensor digitorum longus.
Instructions to person:	Point your toes up and out.

3. Palpate pulses:

   A. Posterior tibial artery—with the ankle inverted to relax the reticulum, palpate this pulse in the groove between the posterior distal end of the medial malleolus and the Achilles tendon. Invert the ankle to relax the reticulum. See Figure 7-10.

   B. Dorsal pedis artery—place your fingers between the bases of the great toe and second toe, then trace that line straight up the foot to the dorsal-most prominence of the navicular bone. See Figure 7-9.

4. Perform the motions of the ankle and foot joint with your partner.

   A. Perform a motion and have your partner name the motion you performed.

   B. Your partner states a motion and then you perform that motion.

5. Observe the amount of motion available at each joint. For each of the motions available at each joint, estimate the degrees of motion available by checking the box in the table below that *most closely* describes that amount of motion. (Do not measure with a goniometer.)

Motions	0°–45°	46°–90°	91°–135°	136°–180°
Dorsiflexion				
Plantar flexion				
MTP flexion				
MTP extension				
MTP abduction of the great toe				

6. Passively move your partner through the available range of motion of the ankle joint, noting end feel. If possible, repeat with several people. Review pre-lab worksheet Question 12 for the normal end feel.

   A. Is your partner's end feel consistent with normal end feel?

   _____

   B. What structures create the end feel for this joint?

   _____

7. With your partner sitting with her or his knee flexed, try to passively dorsiflex your partner's ankle. With your partner long sitting with her or his knee extended, passively flex the ankle. In which position did your partner have the most dorsiflexion ROM? Why?

   _____

   _____

   _____

   _____

8. Use a disarticulated skeleton or anatomical model of the ankle joint and apply the rules of joint arthrokinematics and the concave-convex rule to perform the following exercises.

   A. Move the talus on the tibia in all planes of motion.

   B. Observe the movement of the distal bone on the proximal bone. Circle the motions that you observed.

   Roll   Spin   Glide

   C. Observe the movement of the distal end of the tibia in relation to the movement of the proximal end of the tibia as you move the tibia on the talus.

   Does the distal end of the tibia move in the _____ same direction or _____ opposite direction of the proximal end of the tibia?

9. Stand with your back no more than 6 inches from a wall. Lean backward from your ankles until your shoulders touch the wall. Return to standing erect.

   A. What ankle motion allows you to lean backward?

   _____

   B. Which ankle muscle(s) control the movement as you lean backward?

   _____

   C. What type of muscle contraction controls the motion of leaning backward?

   _____

   D. What ankle motion allows you to return to an erect standing position?

   _____

   E. Which ankle muscle(s) control the return to erect standing motion?

   _____

   F. What type of muscle contraction controls the return to erect standing motion?

   _____

   G. What term is used to describe muscle action that occurs when the origin moves rather than the insertion?

   _____

10. The anatomical axes of the tibia and calcaneus may form a very slight angle. This angle is measured by aligning a goniometer over the posterior midline of the tibia and calcaneus with the pivot at the ankle joint.

    • Calcaneal varus is a decreased angle resulting in the calcaneus appearing to be inverted.

    • Calcaneal valgus is an increased angle resulting in the calcaneus appearing to be everted.

    A. Observe your partner's tibial calcaneal angle in the standing position.

    B. Is the observed angle:
    _____ Normal _____ Decreased
    _____ Increased

   C. Are the right and left angles the
   _____ Same _____ Different

   D. Observe the heels of your partner's shoes for the part of the heel that is most worn. Does this correlate with the position of the calcaneus?

   _____

   _____

11. Dip the sole of one foot in a tub of water and then briefly step on a piece of paper (e.g., a paper towel). Observe the watermark your foot left on the paper.

    A. Describe the parts of your foot that contacted the supporting surface.

    _____

    B. Does the watermark indicate your foot is in
    _____ pes cavus? _____ pes planus?

12. Analyze the activity of the right ankle when descending stairs, leading with the left foot. Start facing down the stairs with both feet on the top step. Lower your left foot to the next lower stair.

    A. What motion is your right ankle performing?
    _____

    B. Which major muscle group is the agonist?
    _____

    C. Is the agonist performing a concentric or an eccentric contraction? _____

    D. Is this an open or closed kinetic chain activity?
    _____

13. Analyze the activity of the right ankle when ascending stairs, leading with the right foot. Start facing up the stairs with both feet at the bottom step. Place your right foot on the first stair and lift your body up using the right leg.

    A. Which motion is your right ankle performing?
    _____

    B. Which major muscle group is the agonist?
    _____

    C. Is the agonist performing a concentric or an eccentric contraction? _____

14. **Functional activity analysis:**

In each chapter on the lower extremity, you will be analyzing the activity of moving from sitting to standing, and the reverse motion of moving from standing to sitting. Perform these activities and then analyze how the subject in Figures 20-28 through 20-32 performed those activities.

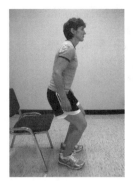

FIGURE 20-31 Midposition.

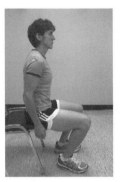

FIGURE 20-28 Starting position to assume standing.

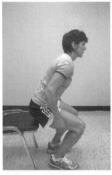

FIGURE 20-29 Initiating standing.

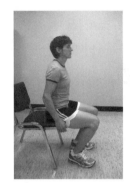

FIGURE 20-32 Ending position for sitting.

A. Describe the positions of the ankle when the subject is:

1) moving from sitting to standing. _____

_____

2) moving from standing to sitting. _____

_____

B. Which muscle groups are acting as prime movers in the following motions?

1) Moving from sitting to standing _____

_____

2) Moving from standing to sitting _____

_____

C. Describe the types of muscle contractions being used in the following motions:

1) Moving from sitting to standing _____

_____

2) Moving from standing to sitting _____

_____

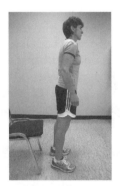

FIGURE 20-30 Ending position for standing. Starting position for sitting.

D. Explain your answers to part C.

1) Moving from sitting to standing _____

_____

2) Moving from standing to sitting _____

_____

15. Place your right index finger on your partner's left medial malleolus and your left index finger on the left lateral malleolus. Keep your fingers parallel to the floor.

A. Describe the orientation of the malleoli in relation to one another.

_____

_____

_____

B. Your fingers are representing the axis for which joint?

_____

16. Using a skin pencil or colored yarn, follow the paths of the major nerves that serve the ankle joint muscles.

Nerves to trace:
- Sciatic
- Tibial
- Common peroneal
- Superficial peroneal
- Deep peroneal

■ ■ ■ Post-Lab Questions

Student's Name _____

Date Due _____

After you have completed the Worksheets and Lab Activities, answer the following questions without using your book or notes. When finished, check your answers.

1. List the motions and prime movers for each of the following joints.

Joints	Motions	Muscles
Ankle		
Subtalar		
Metatarsophalangeal of great toe		

2. List the attachments for the following ankle and foot ligaments.

Ligament	Proximal Attachments	Distal Attachments
Deltoid		
Spring		
Lateral		
Long plantar		

3. For the following ankle and foot ligaments, give the function.

Ligament	Function
Deltoid	
Lateral	
Long plantar	
Plantar aponeurosis	

4. Indicate the relationship of the peroneal muscles' tendons to the lateral malleolus.

Muscle	Anterior	Posterior
Peroneus longus		
Peroneus brevis		
Peroneus tertius		

5. In general, which nerves innervate the following muscle groups?

Muscle Group	Nerve
Dorsiflexors	
Plantar flexors	
Evertors	

6. Starting at the anterior medial aspect of the ankle, name in order the muscles/tendons that cross the ankle as you move laterally around the ankle joint.

_____

_____

_____

7. What is the effect of toe extension on the longitudinal arches of the foot?

_____

_____

8. Give the keystone bone for the arches of the foot.

Arch	Keystone Bone
Medial longitudinal	
Lateral longitudinal	
Transverse	

9. List the bones that make up each of the following parts of the foot.

Foot Part	Bones
Hindfoot	
Midfoot	
Forefoot	

10. Which nerve is superficial at the head of the fibula?

_____

11. Give the prime movers and the muscles that must act to neutralize undesired motions when only the motion listed is to be performed.

Motion	Prime Mover	What Motion Needs to Be Neutralized?	Neutralizer
Dorsiflexion			
Inversion			
Eversion			

12. Why might a person have less ankle dorsiflexion when the knee is extended?

13. The sustentaculum tali is located on which bone?

14. What is the function of the sustentaculum tali?

15. Name the divisions of the sciatic nerve as it passes from the thigh to the foot.

16. List the muscles in each of the following groups.

Muscle Group	Muscles
Superficial posterior	
Deep posterior	
Anterior	

Clinical Kinesiology and
Anatomy of the Body

Posture

■ ■ ■ Pre-Lab Worksheets

Student's Name _____

Date Due _____

Complete the following questions prior to the lab class.

1. Define the following terms:

Primary curve:

_____

_____

Secondary curves:

_____

_____

Antigravity muscles:

_____

_____

Postural sway:

_____

_____

2. For the following landmarks, when performing a standing postural assessment from the lateral view, check the box where the plumb line should be in relation to the body.

Landmark	Anterior	Posterior	Through
Ear			
Tip of the acromion			
Thoracic spine			
Lumbar spine			
Hip			
Knee			
Ankle			

3. View Figure 21-1, then indicate in the following table whether the anterior and posterior curves are concave or convex.

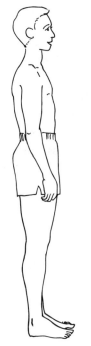

FIGURE 21-1 Anterior and posterior curves.

Spine Region	Posterior Curve	Anterior Curve
Cervical		
Thoracic		
Lumbar		
Sacral		

4. In Figures 21-2, 21-3, and 21-4, identify the positions of the pelvis as anterior tilt, neutral, or posterior tilt.

5. Name the muscle groups that contract concentrically to produce anterior and posterior pelvic tilts.

Position	Muscle Groups
Anterior pelvic tilt	
Posterior pelvic tilt	

6. For a person with a fixed anterior or posterior tilt, identify the muscles that are shortened and those that are lengthened.

Position	Shortened	Lengthened
Anterior pelvic tilt		
Posterior pelvic tilt		

7. In the supine position, a person has an excessive lumbar lordosis. Does this person most likely have _____ an anterior or _____ a posterior pelvic tilt?

8. Standing with good posture, which muscle groups are responsible for maintaining pelvic alignment in the following planes?

Plane	Muscle Groups
Sagittal	
Frontal	
Transverse	

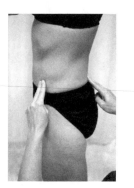

FIGURE 21-2 Examining pelvic tilt.

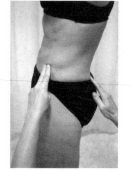

FIGURE 21-3 Examining pelvic tilt.

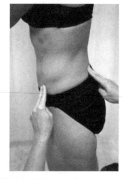

FIGURE 21-4 Examining pelvic tilt.

■ ■ ■ Lab Activities

Student's Name _____

Date Due _____

1. Make a chart on the board, list each class member by some identifying code, and indicate whether the classmate is right- or left-handed.
   - Observe your partner from the posterior view and determine if either the right or left shoulder is higher.
   - Enter the information on the chart on the board.
   - When all have entered their data, analyze the data for any correlation between shoulder position and hand dominance.

   _____

   _____

   _____

2. Perform an observation of posture. Work in groups of three.
   - Suspend a string with a weight (plumb line) from the ceiling.
   - In all views, position the subject's feet 2 to 4 inches apart, with the heels even and the toes pointing slightly outward, close to the plumb line but not so close that they will touch the plumb line when they sway.
   - Align the feet with the plumb line. In the anterior and posterior views, the plumb line should divide the space between the feet evenly. In the side view, the plumb line should be about 2 inches in front of the lateral malleolus.
   - The forms that follow can be used to record your observations.
   - Each member of the group is to be the subject, the lead observer, and the assistant observer during this activity.
   - Observe your partner's posture from all views using a plumb line.
   - Do not get too detailed and do not take too long. Some individuals become faint from standing still for a long time due to pooling of blood. Work in a timely manner and provide the subject with opportunities to walk around between views.

Anterior View: Normal Alignment

Feet	Slight outward toeing
Ankles	Normal arch
Knees	Level Knock-kneed/bowed
Legs	Slightly apart
Iliac crest (see Fig. 17-3)	Level
Sternum	Centered in midline
Shoulders	Level **FIGURE 21-5** Identifying height of shoulders.
Head	Extended Level

Posterior View: Normal Alignment

Ankles	Calcaneus straight Calcaneus inverted/everted
Knees	Level Knock-kneed/bowed
Hips (see Fig. 17-4)	PSIS level
Spinous processes	Centered in midline
Scapula	Level No winging present
Shoulders	Level
Head	Extended Level

Lateral View: Normal Alignment Relative to Plumb Line

_____ Right _____ Left

Ankles	Slightly anterior to lateral malleolus Joint in neutral position
Knees	Slightly posterior to patella Joint in extension
Hips	Through greater trochanter
Pelvis	Level (ASIS and pubic symphysis parallel vertically)
Lumbar spine	Lordotic Flat
Thoracic spine	Kyphotic Flat
Acromion process	Through tip of acromion
Ear	Through earlobe

3. Position your partner in a sitting position in the ways described here, and observe what happens to his or her posture.

   • For a person sitting for long periods, whether in a wheelchair or a desk chair, proper fit of the chair is important. A chair seat that is too wide or too short, too high or too low interferes with a person's ability to maintain good sitting alignment.

   • Chairs such as student desk chairs, office chairs, and sofa chairs can be used in these activities. For chairs without armrests, place empty chairs on either side of your partner with pillows or boxes to simulate armrests. Place a footstool or books of varying thickness on the floor in front of the chair to simulate footrests. Various sizes of wheelchairs can be used with these activities.

   A. Have your partner sit in a chair that is much wider than her or him. When using a chair without armrests, place the simulated armrests 6 inches to the side away from your partner's hips. Instruct your partner to lean on one armrest. Describe the posture of your partner's spine.

   _____

   B. Have your partner sit in a chair that is narrower than her or him. To simulate armrests, place boxes or pillows touching your patient. What bony landmark(s) will be under excessive pressure in this sitting posture?

   _____

   C. With your partner in a sitting position, vary the height of the seat and footrests to achieve the following positions.

   1) The hips and knees are at 90 degrees of flexion, and the feet are flat on a supporting surface.

   2) Adjust a footstool so the hips are in approximately 110 degrees of flexion, the knees are at 90 degrees of flexion, and the feet are flat on a supporting surface.

   3) Adjust the height of the seat so that your partner's feet barely reach the floor.

   What postural adjustment does your partner make in the second and third positions compared to the first position?

   _____

   _____

   Which bony landmark(s) will be under more pressure in the second and third positions?

   _____

   _____

4. Proper alignment in the supine position includes the shoulder girdle and pelvic girdle parallel to each other and centered.

   • Observe your partner in the supine position in proper alignment.

   • Next, have your partner move his or her buttock to the left and maintain the shifted position.

   Describe the alignment of the spine in the new position in terms of concavity. What is the pathological term for this alignment?

   _____

5. With your partner standing, place a block under the left leg to simulate a short right leg. The block should be high enough that the person can stand upright with the knee extended, but just barely so. Have the person remain standing on the block for a couple minutes, then analyze the posture.

   A. Is the head in the midline? _____

   B. If not, to which side is it positioned? _____

   C. Are the shoulders level? If not, which side is higher? _____

   D. Are the iliac crests level? If not, which side is higher? _____

   E. Is the pelvis in a neutral tilt? If not, is it in an _____ anterior or _____ posterior tilt position?

   F. Is the vertebral column curved in a lateral direction? If so, which side is concave?

   _____

6. Have your partner sit in front of a computer screen (or simulation of one).

   • First, assume a position of good posture.

   • Next, have the person slouch. Notice the change in position.

   A. What has changed with the head? _____

   B. What has changed with the cervical spine?

   _____

   C. What has changed with the thoracic spine?

   _____

   D. What has changed with the lumbar spine?

   _____

   E. What has changed with the pelvis?

   _____

■ ■ ■ Post-Lab Questions

Student's Name _____

Date Due _____

After you have completed the worksheets and lab activities, answer the following questions without using your book or notes. When finished, check your answers.

1. List the normal curve of each segment of the spinal column. Describe the posterior side of the curves.

Spinal Segment	Curve
Cervical	
Thoracic	
Lumbar	
Sacral	
Coccyx	

2. For the postural deviations listed in the following table, check the box(es) that is the best view(s) to use to observe the deviation.

Postural Alignment	Anterior View	Posterior View	Lateral View
Coxa vara			
Genu valgus			
Calcaneal varus			
Uneven shoulders			
Genu recurvatum			

3. Assess the posture in Figure 21-6.

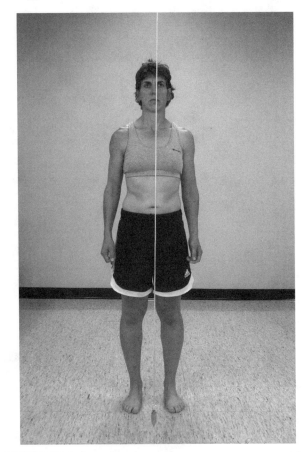

FIGURE 21-6 Anterior view.

Anterior View: Alignment Relative to Plumb Line	
Joint	Location of the Plumb Line in Relation to the Body Part
Feet	
Ankles	
Knees	
Legs	
Hips	
Sternum	
Shoulders	
Head	

4. Examine the posture in Figure 21-7.

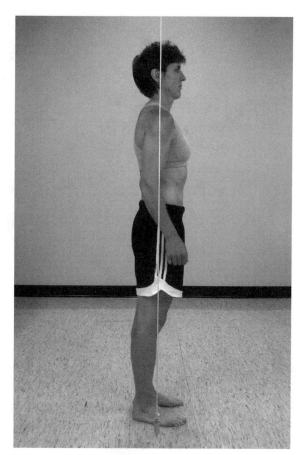

FIGURE 21-7 Right lateral view.

Right Lateral View: Alignment Relative to Plumb Line

Joint	Location of the Plumb Line in Relation to the Body Part
Ankles	
Knees	
Hips	
Pelvis	
Lumbar spine	
Thoracic spine	
Acromion process	
Ear	

5. A posture examination indicates which muscles or structures should be further examined to determine their strength or length. For each of the following postural deviations, list two structures that should be examined and for what purpose.

Postural Alignment	Structure to Examine	Purpose for Examination
Lack of full knee extension		
Anterior pelvic tilt		
Left iliac crest lower than right iliac crest		

Gait

■ ■ ■ An Introduction

The positions of the hip, knee, ankle, and toes have been described for each phase of gait for the Rancho Los Amigos (RLA) approach to gait assessment. These positions are as follows:

Initial Contact		Preswing	
Hip:	25° flexion	Hip:	0°
Knee:	0°	Knee:	40° flexion
Ankle:	0°	Ankle:	20° plantar flexion
Toes:	0°	Toes:	60° MTP extension
Loading Response		**Initial Swing**	
Hip:	25° flexion	Hip:	15° flexion
Knee:	15° flexion	Knee:	60° flexion
Ankle:	10° plantar flexion	Ankle:	10° plantar flexion
Toes:	0°	Toes:	0°
Midstance		**Midswing**	
Hip:	0°	Hip:	25° flexion
Knee:	0°	Knee:	25° flexion
Ankle:	5° dorsiflexion	Ankle:	0°
Toes:	0°	Toes:	0°
Terminal Stance		**Terminal Swing**	
Hip:	20° hyperextension	Hip:	25° flexion
Knee:	0°	Knee:	0°
Ankle:	10° dorsiflexion	Ankle:	0°
Toes:	30° MTP extension	Toes:	0°

Source: Observational Gait Analysis Handbook. The Pathokinesiology Service and the Physical Therapy Department of Rancho Los Amigos Medical Center, Downey, CA, 1993.

■ ■ ■ **Pre-Lab Worksheets** _____

Student's Name _____

Date Due _____

Complete the following questions prior to the lab class.

1. A. A line drawn between successive midpoints of heel strike would reveal what about a person's walking base? _____

   B. What is highest at midstance and lowest at heel strike? _____

   C. The number of steps taken per minute is called? _____

   D. As the center of gravity shifts from side to side during walking, there are equal amounts of

   _____ .

2. A. In what way are Trendelenburg sign and Trendelenburg gait similar?

   _____

   B. In what way are Trendelenburg sign and Trendelenburg gait different?

   _____

   _____

3. Match the following term(s) with the appropriate description:

   _____ Occurs during swing phase   A. Single leg support, midstance

   _____ Body weight shifts, allowing one leg to swing   B. Weight acceptance, heel strike

   _____ Stance phase   C. Leg advancement

4. Match the description with the appropriate period of the gait cycle.

   _____ Occurs during approximately 40% of the gait cycle   A. Nonsupport

   _____ Center of gravity is the lowest point   B. Single-leg support

   _____ Does not occur in walking   C. Double-leg support

5. Match the following descriptions with the appropriate period or point of the gait cycle.

   _____ Between end of toe-off and end of acceleration   A. Initial contact

   _____ Between end of foot flat and end of midstance   B. Foot flat

   _____ Between end of midstance and end of heel-off   C. Midstance

   _____ The leg swung as far forward as it is going to   D. Terminal stance

   _____ Body weight begins to shift onto stance leg   E. Preswing

   _____ Between end of acceleration and end of midswing   F. Initial swing

   _____ Just before and including when toes leave ground   G. Midswing

   _____ Entire foot is in contact with the ground   H. Deceleration

6. Using both traditional terminology and RLA terminology, list in order of occurrence the components of the gait cycle.

Traditional	RLA
STANCE	*STANCE*
Heel strike	Initial contact
	XX—No comparable term

Traditional	RLA
SWING	*SWING*

7. Match the following terms and definitions.

_____ Distance between heel strike of one foot and heel strike of the other foot   A. Stance phase

_____ Side-to-side distance between heels   B. Stride length

_____ Distance between heel strike of one foot and heel strike of the same foot   C. Step width

_____ That part of the gait cycle when the foot is in contact with the ground   D. Swing phase

_____ That part of the gait cycle when the foot is not in contact with the ground   E. Step length

8. For each phase of the gait cycle, the amount of range of motion at the hip, knee, and ankle varies. Deviation from the normal range is one of the causes of increased energy cost during walking. For each joint at each phase of the gait cycle, indicate the approximate normal range of motion.

Initial Contact

Joint	ROM
Hip	
Knee	
Ankle	
Toes	

Loading Response

Joint	ROM
Hip	
Knee	
Ankle	
Toes	

Midstance

Joint	ROM
Hip	
Knee	
Ankle	
Toes	

Terminal Stance

Joint	ROM
Hip	
Knee	
Ankle	
Toes	

Preswing

Joint	ROM
Hip	
Knee	
Ankle	
Toes	

Initial Swing

Joint	ROM
Hip	
Knee	
Ankle	
Toes	

Midswing

Joint	ROM
Hip	
Knee	
Ankle	
Toes	

Terminal Swing

Joint	ROM
Hip	
Knee	
Ankle	
Toes	

9. Joint movement during gait is produced by muscle contractions, gravity, and joint response in a closed-kinetic chain. Determining the direction of joint movement, within a phase and from one phase of gait to the next, is necessary to analyze which muscles are working and what type of contraction a muscle is performing. For each phase of the gait cycle, indicate:

A. The position (or motion) that is occurring at each joint.

B. Briefly describe what is happening. Examples include unchanged, slight flexion from full extension, and increasing dorsiflexion.

Initial Contact (From Terminal Swing)

Joint	Position	Description
Hip		
Knee		
Ankle		

Loading Response (From Initial Contact)

Joint	Position	Description
Hip		
Knee		
Ankle		

Midstance (From Loading Response)

Joint	Position	Description
Hip		
Knee		
Ankle		

Terminal Stance (From Midstance)

Joint	Position	Description
Hip		
Knee		
Ankle		

Preswing (From Terminal Stance)

Joint	Position	Description
Hip		
Knee		
Ankle		

Initial Swing (From Preswing)

Joint	Position	Description
Hip		
Knee		
Ankle		

Midswing (From Midswing)

Joint	Position	Description
Hip		
Knee		
Ankle		

Terminal Swing (From Initial Swing)

Joint	Position	Description
Hip		
Knee		
Ankle		

10. In Figure 22-1, identify the phases of the gait cycle for each leg.

    Right leg: _____

    Left leg: _____

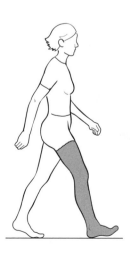

FIGURE 22-1

11. Regarding the end of the period in Figure 22-2, what is the position of the right ankle and left knee in terms of ROM?

    Right ankle: _____ Left knee: _____

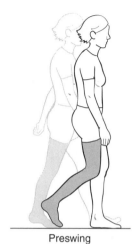
Preswing

FIGURE 22-2 Preswing period (RLA). The lighter tone shows the beginning and the darker tone shows the end of this period.

12. In Figure 22-3, identify which muscle(s) are controlling the right knee and left ankle and what type of contractions are being performed.

    _____

    _____

    _____

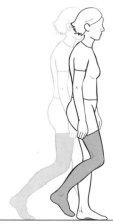

FIGURE 22-3 Initial swing period (RLA). The lighter tone shows the beginning and the darker tone shows the ending of this period.

■ ■ ■ Lab Activities

Student's Name _____

Date Due _____

1. As a class, demonstrate each phase of the gait cycle.

2. Step length, stride length, and step width can be measured using simple methods. One method is:

   A. Tape about a 10-foot length of absorbent paper on the floor with a chair placed at one end.

   B. The subject dips the bottoms of bare feet in water and walks with a normal gait and cadence. One observer records the time to walk from the first heel strike to the last heel strike on the paper.

   C. Place a mark at and label each heel strike as either right or left foot.

   D. Measure the distances between heel strikes of the same foot, heel strikes of opposite feet, and the width between heel strikes of opposite feet.

   E. Count the number of strides and use the time walked to determine the speed of the gait.

3. Observe the gait of your partners from the front, side, and back. This is most easily done using a treadmill. If one is not available, arrange an area large enough so the subject is able to walk at normal speed and the observers have sufficient room to observe and move as needed to watch from the front, back, and each side. When viewing from the side, the observers should walk sideways to be able to watch the subject directly as he or she walks.

   A. Initial observations should be of the "whole person" as the individual walks. Note speed and any unusual gait patterns.

   B. Observe each joint through the full cycle of gait, identifying the phase.

   C. Observe each joint through the full cycle to determine the ROM. Make note of any ROM at any joint that is not normal. On the following form, indicate the phase of the gait cycle and if the ROM is less than normal (−), greater than normal (+), or normal (N).

Initial Contact

Joint	ROM
Hip	
Knee	
Ankle	
Toes	

Loading Response

Joint	ROM
Hip	
Knee	
Ankle	
Toes	

Midstance

Joint	ROM
Hip	
Knee	
Ankle	
Toes	

Terminal Stance

Joint	ROM
Hip	
Knee	
Ankle	
Toes	

Preswing

Joint	ROM
Hip	
Knee	
Ankle	
Toes	

Midswing

Joint	ROM
Hip	
Knee	
Ankle	
Toes	

Initial Swing

Joint	ROM
Hip	
Knee	
Ankle	
Toes	

Terminal Swing

Joint	ROM
Hip	
Knee	
Ankle	
Toes	

4. Being able to identify typical gait deviations is important. Imitating gait deviations is one way to learn to identify atypical gait patterns and the energy requirements that result. Imitate the following gait deviations and observe your partner imitating those gait deviations.

General Cause of Abnormal Gait	Description of Resulting Abnormal Gait
Gluteus maximus weakness	Compensated by: Quickly shifting the trunk posteriorly at heel strike (initial contact) on the side of the weak gluteus maximus so COG is posterior to axis of hip joint.
Gluteus medius weakness	Compensated by: Shifting the trunk over the side of the weak gluteus medius during stance.
Quadriceps weakness	Compensated by: At heel strike (initial contact and loading response) on the side of the weakness, leaning body forward so COG is anterior to axis of knee joint. Another method is to use the ipsilateral hand to hold the knee in extension during stance.
Hamstring weakness	Uncompensated: Excessive or fast extension of the knee during deceleration (terminal swing).

General Cause of Abnormal Gait	Description of Resulting Abnormal Gait
Ankle dorsiflexor weakness	Uncompensated: Toes strike ground first instead of the heel (equinus gait). Strength permits heel strike (initial contact) to occur but not controlled movement to foot flat (loading response), which results in foot slap. During swing phase, the ankle remains in plantar flexion (drop foot). Compensated by: Excessive hip flexion (steppage gait).
Triceps surae group weakness	Uncompensated: No heel rise or push-off, resulting in a shortened step length on the unaffected side.
Diffuse weakness of many muscle groups	Compensated by: Waddling gait; shoulders posterior to hips and lateral shift to weight-bearing side. Little pelvic motion. To advance a leg, the entire side of the body swings forward. Excessive hip flexion may be needed because of ankle dorsiflexor weakness.
Hip flexion contracture	Compensated by: The trunk leans forward during stance phase on the involved side.
Fused hip	Compensated by: Increased motion of the lumbar spine and pelvis.
Knee flexion contracture	Compensated by: Excessive dorsiflexion during midstance and an early heel rise during push-off (terminal stance). Short step length on unaffected side.
Knee fused in extension	Compensated by: 1. Toe rise (vaulting) of uninvolved side during stance to allow involved side to clear during midswing (vaulting gait). 2. Hip hike on the involved side during swing. 3. Swing leg out to side (circumducted gait).
Triceps surae contracture: Ankle in plantar flexion	Uncompensated: Knee forced into excessive extension during midstance; unable to progress tibia over foot from midstance on through rest of stance phase.
Ankle fusion: Triple arthrodesis	Uncompensated: Loss of ankle pronation and supination makes walking on uneven surfaces difficult; limited ankle dorsiflexion and plantar flexion; short stride length.
Ataxic gait	Uncompensated: Poor balance, uneven, jerky, exaggerated movements. Compensated by: Wide base of support.
Scissors gait	Uncompensated: Excessive adduction and lateral body shift during swing phase; narrow base.
Crouch gait	Uncompensated: Increased lumbar lordosis; anterior pelvic tilt; excessive hip flexion, adduction, and medial rotation; excessive knee flexion; ankles dorsi flexed. Compensated by: Excessive arm movement.
Antalgic gait	Compensated by: Short stance phase on involved side results in rapid and short step length of the uninvolved side. May alter arm swing.

5. In a group, observe what happens to the components of gait as an individual varies cadence from very slow to very fast (do not run). Describe the changes you observe.

_____

_____

_____

6. In a group, observe what happens to the components of gait when an individual uses an assistive device such as a cane, a walker, or a sling on one arm. Describe how the gait changes in each situation.

Cane: _____

_____

Walker: _____

_____

Sling: _____

_____

■ ■ ■ Post-Lab Questions

Student's Name _____

Date Due _____

After you have completed the worksheets and lab activities, answer the following questions without using your book or notes. When finished, check your answers.

1. Identify the following descriptions of gait phases by giving the traditional terminology and the RLA terminology.

Description of Gait Phase	Traditional Terminology	Rancho Los Amigos Terminology
Body weight shock is absorbed.		
Hip is at maximum flexion.		
Hip is hyperextended and knee is starting to flex.		
The foot strikes the ground.		
Period of single limb support		
Leg is behind body and moving forward.		
Dorsiflexors contract eccentrically.		
Body passes over weight-bearing leg.		
Hamstrings contract eccentrically.		
Toes are in extreme hyperextension.		

2. Indicate the direction of movement (flexing or extending) at the following joints in the phases of gait given.

   A. Heel strike to foot flat—initial contact to loading response

   Knee: _____

   Ankle: _____

   B. Foot flat to midstance—loading response to midstance

   Hip: _____

   Ankle: _____

   C. Heel-off to toe-off-terminal stance to preswing

   Knee: _____

   Ankle: _____

   D. Acceleration to midswing-initial swing to midswing

   Hip: _____

   Knee: _____

3. In which phases of gait do the following motions occur?

   A. Hip flexion: _____

   B. Knee extension: _____

   C. Ankle dorsiflexion: _____